THE HANDS-ON
APPROACH

The Ultimate Guide To Getting Rid Of Nagging Hand and
Shoulder Problems Without Pills, Injections, and Surgery

HOANG TRAN

Publisher: Hoang Tran, Hands-On Therapy Services 7902 NW 36th St Ste 207 Doral, FL 33166

ISBN: 9781795446419
Imprint: Independently published

Dedication

To my family - Ryan, Connor, and especially Hailey who helped create chapter titles. And my father-in-law Richard, forced out of retirement to help edit this book.

To my clients for trusting in Hands-On Therapy Services to provide you with an experience unlike any other and the solution you were looking for.

Success stories

A few success stories from our clients with hand and shoulder problems whether they were avoiding surgery or getting help after surgery.

Vanessa -
"I highly recommend Hands On Therapy Services Inc. to anyone suffering from any upper extremities injury... .I had been suffering from Frozen Shoulder for 5 months...I was able to regain 85% mobility while also concentrating on strength training. Ask Hoang anything about your condition and she will give you a full explanation while demonstrating what you can do at home to help your rehab... Give them a call and welcome your health back!!!!

Mary
...I have been coming (to Hands on Therapy Services) for at least 4-5 month, the relief I feel has been amazing. I cannot tell you...I was scared to death of having...surgery, so I thought this I will try and see how it works.

Shirley
"...I couldn't turn in bed I couldn't sleep...now I am out there playing golf, which I couldn't play all the time, I feel so much stronger and relax on my shoulders."

Cherlyn
"The staff is very professional...the best to go to if you are having problems or surgery on your hands, shoulders or arms. She could also be a comedian because if you walk in feeling sad or down about anything, she will have you smiling and laughing in no time."

Kip
"The staff is very caring and go out of their way to make you feel comfortable. I am so happy that we chose them for my sons hand injury. They not only cared for his wound and gave...therapy for his hand, they helped an old shoulder injury that he had when he was 17 years old."

Linda
"Shoulder pain was making my golf game less than enjoyable, but I wasn't about to stop playing golf. On the advice of a friend, I paid a visit to Hoang Tran at Hands On Therapy Services. A few visits later, the shoulder pain had lessened and work on hips and lower body helped to rejuvenate my golf swing and make it a lot more fun again."

Laynys
"I felt so comfortable here. They made me feel welcome since the moment I called..."

Lily
"My boyfriend had a terrible elbow dislocated and went almost under surgery...His surgeon recommended Hoang and Hands-on Therapy Services and he has been going under therapy...and the recovery has been amazing...he will be able to kitesurf again very soon"

T Rouette
"Nothing, but good things to say about Hands on Therapy Services! The staff is warm and welcoming and provided personalized attention and the knowledgeable insight I needed for long term care."

Ahmad

My experience at Hands On Therapy has been superb. After going through three occupational therapy offices, I had plateaued until I became a patient at Hands On. My injury and needs were given a tailored approach and the therapy I received was methodological and progressed according to my needs. The time dedicated to each patient and the expertise in hand and arm rehabilitation at Hands On has surpassed any other therapy experience that I have had. I believe that I would not have progressed beyond that plateau and gained the functionality and flexibility that I now have had I not been a patient at Hands On. I would recommend Hands On Therapy as a first choice to anyone in need of occupational therapy.

Rocio

My experience at Hands on Therapy Services has been excellent.... helped me be pain free in just a few visits and she is training me to maintain myself well balanced. I have never felt so understood while explaining my conditions and I really feel that I am healing from the inside out, the root of my problems, and not covering up the symptoms with painful injections or surgery as doctors have recommended me in the past. The "girls", as we call the staff, are just so sweet and always prompt to assist and pamper me during my sessions and even after working hours, when they have guided me through an emergency.

Lina

Very professional and friendly place, I truly love the one on one treatment I'm receiving. I highly recommend it for someone that needs a great therapist. You will not be disappointed.

Contents

About the Author

Hoang Tran is an Occupational Therapist and Certified Hand Therapist. She is the owner of Hands-on Therapy Services in Doral (Miami), FL, where she works with people 40+ to stay active, pain free, and avoid pills, injections, and surgery. She particularly specializes in helping those with arm and hand injuries.

Raised right here in Miami, she returned home after attending University of Florida. After almost 20 years helping patients in big hospital settings, she set forth to create a private clinic where people can come to get the kind experience she would want for her own family and friends.

In her spare time, Hoang is an adjunct professor in the Occupational Therapy Department at Barry University in Miami Shores, teaches Continuing Education courses for licensed Occupational Therapists, and mentors other occupational therapists who are training to become Certified Hand Therapists. When not at the clinic or teaching, she can be found hanging out with her husband and two kids or having some girl time with her friends.

Introduction

"I can't tell you exactly when I started feeling that way because it's been so long. I don't even remember a time when I woke up without feeling really tight and achy around my neck and shoulders, and sometimes my hands feel so numb."

Does this story sound similar to yours? I hear stories like this all the time from people who suffer from arm and hand pain.

When asked why she waited so long to get help, her response rang similar to other stories I've heard. Her arm and hand pain is not BAD pain. "It doesn't really stop me from doing anything...it's just that I know when I do certain things I will have more pain later. I thought it would go away because it always has before."

The problems of arm and hand pain may have you thinking that they don't "stop" you from doing anything. They just slow you down a little sometimes. You may not even notice it at first, but maybe the pain has kept you from enjoying yoga classes or going to the gym because of how you will feel later. Maybe you don't offer to entertain friends as much because you know all the work it requires will hurt when they are gone.

Little by little, although it doesn't seem like the arm and hand problems have stopped you from doing anything, they have robbed you of truly enjoying many things you loved to do before the aches and pains and worry about what could be wrong.

Does it seem impossible that you could get rid of arm and hand problems? If you are someone who is worried, has suffered for a long time, and is hopeless of ever finding a solution, keep reading! I've written this book just for you! I want to offer you hope that there are real solutions to your pain that don't involve pills, injections, or surgery.

Or if you have had an accident that required surgery, I understand your concern over what you need to do now as well the impact on your future. That's exactly what one of our client's mom was thinking. At 12 years old, he had major surgery on his hand. "What does he need to do now to be able to start moving and using his hand again?" The real concern was his potential to play basketball or even just with other kids on the playground. And what about his future? Would his hand ever get back to normal or would it hinder his future career? Would he be able to play with the children he hasn't even had yet? Every mom of a 12 or 20 or 30 year old has had those concerns.

If you had arm or hand surgery and wonder what is possible, then continue reading. This book is for you as well. I've worked with many clients over the years who did not initially get the answers or results they had hoped for and wondered, "could there more to my recovery?" The answer is YES!

This book is full of stories about people just like you and me. They all had arm and hand problems, injuries, and worries, and they all found a solution that worked. I've included many of my tips, advice, and ways for you to get started if you have questions and worries about your arm and hand problems. These are real tips and solutions that have worked for my clients, and I want to share them with you, so that you can know all the possibilities to finally get your full life back.

So flip to whatever point in this book speaks to your situation. I'll meet you where you need me most. See you there!

Chapter 1

Why Do Anything About
Hand & Arm Problems?

Widely held false beliefs

ARE YOU SOMEONE who is living with arm and hand problems but don't think they are serious right now (and are still worried that they might get worse)?

Are you someone who has been living with arm and hand problems for months and even years but feel you can "deal with it" because it will probably go away on its own (although it hasn't)?

Are you thinking that you really do not need to do anything at all because it's not stopping you from doing anything important(or so you think)?

What if everything you've ever been told about your arm and hand problems were wrong?

What if the people who gave you advice didn't have enough information at the time or didn't know the latest treatments to be able to best help you?

What if there were another way?

I would love to help show you the possibilities. My name is Hoang Tran, Occupational Therapist and Certified Hand Therapist. For the past 20 years I have been helping people in Greater Miami just like you who are suffering from arm and hand issues. Whether you know what the problem is or are just not sure – maybe you are starting to feel aches and pains here and there, but it's not yet STOPPING you from doing anything – I can give you clarity on what is going on and what you can do about it.

If you don't want to live a life of constantly taking pills, risking further problems, even surgery, and, more importantly, losing your ability to move and do the simple things you love doing without pain and difficulty, then this book is for you.

So many people I meet have some hand and arm problems. Many of them tell me how it was something that started years ago, got better, and was gone – or so they thought – only to have the problem back again, sometimes worse.

No one wants to be in pain. No one wants to deal with annoying, nagging aches and tightness where you just can't seem to get comfortable no matter the position. Are you waking up at night and must shake out your hands just to get them moving because they feel numb and lifeless? Or getting to the end of the day having so much trouble that you want to do nothing and dread what you will feel like later?

No one wants to be limited in what they can do or stop doing the activities they love. Are you working out but there are one or two exercises that you can't do anymore because you know it will hurt either now or later? Or do you play sports but now must play slower or more cautiously, feeling old and sluggish compared to your friends? If you think it's normal "old age" to have that kind of soreness, tightness, or pain, you are wrong. Limiting yourself and compensating often create other imbalances that can derail you from your fitness goals and active lifestyle.

No one wants to have that nagging worry in the back of his or her mind, either. I know what you are thinking: what will happen if it gets worse? What would it mean? But you don't want to deal with it right now because it's really not that bad yet.

What is stopping you from getting real help? What stories are you telling yourself? What stories are you hearing from other and imagining for yourself?

Ask anyone whether they value their health and wellbeing. They will say yes. Ask anyone whether they value being able to go to sleep easily at night and being able to wake up rested. That's a big fat YES! Ask anyone if they love the freedom to hop in the car to drive themselves or being able to cook a meal or play with their kids and grandkids. Without hesitation, they will tell you how important it is that they are able to do all of that without a worry in their mind.

These things sound simple, something that we all do every day, and it is easy to take them for granted. But all these things are threatened when you have arm and hand problems. I know that it is not always easy to get started in occupational or physical therapy, especially when you are not sure it's going to work. That's why I want to help you clarify the problem and do what actually helps.

There are two different issues.

The first is when the pain or other problems are slow to surface. It's only occasional. Maybe you are reaching and "ouch!" – that one direction hurts your shoulders. But if you stop doing it that way, it won't bother you anymore. Until you do it again. Maybe it's waking up with your hands numb or feeling stiff like pegs. However, if you start moving, they will get a little better. All of this worries you. You wonder if it will get worse and what that will mean. I bet you start to ask your friends and family, and I bet someone in your circle has had these problems too. Most people don't know what to do or where to go. Or maybe they didn't have the best experience when they did go somewhere. What stories are they telling you? Do they value what you value? And what are YOU listening to?

Let me tell you a story. I was in a mom's group on social media. A mom asked me what to do about her hand pain and numbness when she awoke in the morning. She described how much it was bothering her and how often she worried about it. It was more than bothering, however. She was in a lot of pain, not getting much sleep, and having difficulty caring for her growing baby. What should she do? She asked a bunch of strangers in the facebook group for medical advice, as though she was looking for a great place to eat. But she was asking about her health. Imagine all the responses from this large group of more than 10,000 moms. It was overwhelming. She learned of so many different experiences: waiting and the pain went away, wearing hand braces for months or years and still suffering, doing nothing because it's not that bad, recommending this oil and that pill and this service because it's the cheapest and not that service because it's too expensive.

We were glad to help this mom when she decided to take the free information from our website (www.handsots.com). She was able to speak to our specialist, who gave her more clarity on what she needed to do. There is a lot of information out there whether you ask 10,000 people on social media or Google. She even asked her doctor, and because her symptoms were considered "mild," no surgery was recommended. As if she wanted surgery.

My point here is that these people did NOT know her and did NOT know what she VALUED and wanted for herself. But she asked, so they told her. Responses got responses. It's paralyzing sometimes when there are so many options and so much advice, especially medical advice from mostly non-medical people. She didn't know these people, but she was absorbing their advice. They didn't know what

4

she valued and what she was willing to do to get rid of the pain. It's like asking a chef to give heart advice because he had had a heart attack or knew someone who had a heart attack. When you ask someone for medical advice, make sure they get to know you, what you want, and what you value. That way their advice can be thoughtful and meaningful for you, and you can feel confident that you have the information that allows you to make the best decision. Medical doctors are good at medicine and generally will prescribe medicine. Surgeons are great at surgery and most likely will recommend surgery when it's an option. When you go to doctors, they want to help you as fast as possible with what they specialize in – which are pills and surgery. That may not always be what you are looking for.

Occupational Therapists specialize in helping you figure out where you are having difficulty in your everyday activities, work, and hobbies so that we can prescribe ways to get you moving better and without pain. I can help you, as a therapist, if you are someone who is looking for a natural method of getting rid of the pain, one that gets to the root cause of the problem and sets you up for the best chance of not having the problem come back any time soon.

You know that problem is there. You just decided to ignore it because you don't feel it all the time.

A client of mine told me a story I hear too often. His hands have been bothering him for years. He initially claimed it was only a year, but after looking at his hands, he admitted it had been many years. He said he put off getting help because he was busy at work. See, he works for himself and if he didn't work, he couldn't provide for his family. It hurt, but once he was working and moving he didn't feel it as much. Until, of course, later that night when the pain would set in and he would wake up with his hands throbbing. Only after his hands were hurting so much that it was getting in the way of peaceful rest and his daily work did he decide to take care of it. The fear of having to have surgery finally brought him to our clinic. It took him at least three years to make a move. Knowing what he knows now, he

5

says he wishes he hadn't had to suffer for so many years and would have come in sooner had he known what occupational therapy could do to help him remove the pain and avoid surgery.

It's the slow-to-surface type of problems like trigger finger, carpal tunnel syndrome, tennis elbow, or shoulder tendinitis that lead many people to sit for months, even years, without realizing they didn't need to suffer.

The second involves arm and hand injuries after an accident or incident. One day you suddenly can't move or use your arm. You wake up in excruciating pain and can't even lift your arm. Or perhaps there was an accident where you needed surgery to fix a broken bone, but now you can't move that hand. When this happens, there's more urgency for help NOW. There is no option to wait because it is already worse.

Where do you go and what do you do? You turn to your friends and family, you ask your doctor, you ask your insurance. What do they value as compared to what you value when it comes to getting the BEST therapy to regain your arm and hand function, allowing you to do the simplest of things like washing your face, getting dressed, driving or cooking? No one would say, "Let me get the cheapest surgeon to fix my broken hand." You ask, "Who is the best surgeon?" You want the best possible chance to regain function of your arm or hand and to restore the highest quality of life after surgery.

After an accident or surgery, why is everyone only giving you the cheapest option or the closest option when it comes to regaining your life back? Don't you want a full recovery? Everyone that I talk to after an accident wants the chance at 100% recovery. No one tells me it's fine to half-ass it and only get back to 50%. Everyone wants the CHANCE for a full recovery.

Accidents can change your life in an instant. Most people are so shocked by what happened that they are paralyzed about what to do next. There is also an inherent trust in the surgeon and his office because they have been there to help you, especially if they have been kind and supportive. It's hard to look for something outside of that doctor's recommendation. One client told me that he felt compelled to go to the doctor's own therapist because the doctor told him to go there, even though he wasn't making the progress he wanted. To make it worse, he's a surgeon himself who cannot perform surgeries due to his own arm surgery!

Sometimes you are left on your own to find a reputable clinic that specializes in what you need…help after surgery. Most people try to rely on a referral from friends and family, or they call their insurance company, or they look online. That can result in calls upon calls. Eventually you might go to a place to get started, but if your experience is lacking, I urge you to keep looking! It's important to find the specialist who can truly help you reach your full potential for recovery.

If you are someone who has an arm or hand problem that has been slow to progress, such as carpal tunnel, or has suffered an accident that resulted in surgery to fix an elbow fracture, then this book was written for you. If you have any curiosity how you could get real help in improving your chances of living more actively without limits, without pain, without taking pills all the time, without having to consider injections, without unnecessary surgeries, then read on to the next chapter to learn all that is possible.

Chapter 2

Mistakes People Often Make

A S I'M WRITING this book about arm and hand problems, it is after Thanksgiving, a time to be grateful and also to shop black Friday and Cyber Monday deals. My emails are blowing up more than usual with sales for all sorts of things that I probably don't need, and I can't help but notice all the gadgets out there that promise the world, especially when it comes to pain, literally solving it in one fell swoop. I can see why people are drawn to the "fast acting," "take it away for good," and "cures you in X number of days" type of ad campaigns. I saw an ad on social media that promised this ONE gadget would completely cure tennis elbow. I was fascinated. Especially since it was endorsed by a well-known physical therapist.

I'm all in if it were true. I get it. Who doesn't want it to be easy and painless with no effort? Sign me up!

The same can be said about braces and straps. Just wear this "thing" and it will cure all your problems. If it were that easy, no one would have tennis elbow pain.

I know that it is easier to try things like creams, self-massage gadgets of all kinds, braces, and straps. These things are an easy way to start to doing something on your own. They are also easy to purchase and don't require a lot of time and effort (or so you think). There are also a lot of videos that you can find online to help you learn what to do. I think it's a great way to get started. We offer free tips and advice that you can find on our website (www.handsots.com), and we also have a YouTube channel full of free videos (search Hands-On Therapy Services and hit subscribe to get all the latest videos). But many people get stuck there and end up suffering for months or even years.

Are you stuck?

Getting stuck is one of the biggest mistakes that people make when it comes to arm and hand problems. How long are you willing to be stuck? Don't you want to avoid taking pills (weekly or daily) or having injections that don't work? Don't you want to avoid surgery when you can?

The slow-to-show-up type of problem, like carpal tunnel or trigger finger or tennis elbow or shoulder tendinitis, is by far the most common. It's where most people are stuck. Stuck about what to do, about what it could be, and about what solutions are possible.

I encounter this problem every day. Here are a few of the common objections that I hear about when people have arm and hand problems:

It doesn't stop me from doing anything. That is, unless you have had an accident that required surgery, or you woke up and couldn't move your arm or hand. If you suddenly can't write or drive, THAT will make you get help. When it's slow-to-show-up type of problems, you can still do everything. You can wake up and get ready for work, even if it's slow or difficult at first. Get your family ready. Drive to work. Get home. If you can't cook, then why not order out? There's always something that you can do to get around the problem when it comes to everyday independence – until one day when you can't get around it any more. To be honest, it IS stopping you – but you have decided that you can live with limitations. You've decided not to keep going to fitness classes or the gym. Or you've decided not to roughhouse with the kids because it will leave you in more pain. That's why I am trying to help you get unstuck so you won't suffer for so many years only to have something stop you in your tracks. By then it will be extra difficult.

If I rest for a little while it might just go away on its own. Waiting for it to go away on its own? Are you thinking, "if it hurts on one hand and arm, I'll just use the other hand and arm."? Rest can alleviate lots of aches and pain. When you work out and you get sore, working out less intensely can help with the soreness. Sometimes, when you play too hard and become sorer than you expected, taking an over-the-counter painkiller can help alleviate the soreness. Getting in some extra rest is always good. The story is different when you are feeling the need to rest every single time or feeling like you need to take painkillers every day or every week. Honestly, after months and even years, you probably stopped working out or playing that sport or taking that class. But if you could, you would keep going. That is when rest is not the best or only option. You may need additional help.

I want to try to get rid of it on my own. Okay, are you still not ready to go somewhere to fix your pain? You may want to try some home remedies. That's fine! Try essential oils. I use them myself for different things. I like Biofreeze or topical creams, too. I use them with my clients, and I use them with my parents and myself. There's a time and place for them, and they do feel nice if you like that kind of tingling heat on your skin. They do help with mild aches. It also matters how you are massaging the painful areas.

But when do you get professional help from a specialized therapist such as at Hands-On Therapy Services? When it's been months and is still not going away. That's the best time to take care of it because it's not yet stopping you from doing anything. I help people who have been living with problems for years but just didn't think it was

10

important **enough**. Unfortunately, it suddenly turns into a much worse problem, and they are left wondering what happened yesterday. It didn't happen yesterday. Usually, when I dig a little deeper, I find it's been dormant for years, but it wasn't a big problem and didn't stop them from using their arms. Then, one morning, they wake up after sleeping on their side or holding the baby unable to lift their arm.

Are you stuck trying to massage yourself with creams that claim to take away the pain but it's still not better?

Are you stuck using braces but it's only mildly better, though you have been using them for years? I had a guy tell me he had been using his elbow straps for 12 years!

Since these do-it-yourself remedies haven't worked as well as you had hoped, does that leave you feeling hopeless that anything will work? There is hope. I always say that it's great to know what you have already tried, because that gives us a starting point. For one, if you are trying, that means you are invested in your health and well-being! Second, the issue is not always where the problem is. That's why going to a specialist like those at Hands-On Therapy Services is helpful. We can assess the whole way you move in order to find the root cause of the pain.

It's not that important right now. I have other people and things I need to take care of. We only have one body. Two hands and two arms is all we get if we are lucky in this life. It's take care of your body or bust. You can lease a car, you can replace it every three to 10 years if you like, but you cannot replace your body. There are consequences to action as well as **inaction**. I know you take care of the people in your life. The clients I work with tell me all about helping their grown kids with the grandkids, or they tell me about how hard they are working to provide for their family. Not one person tells me they were sitting on their ass doing nothing and being waited on hand and foot. Maybe I am not attracting those people. But you are

11

just as important if not more important to take care of. When you have pain and can't use your arms and hands, you won't be able to help those you love.

More and more people tell me how they are working and looking forward to retirement but that they wished they had done things differently so that they could enjoy their retirement more actively. Some are starting to act now as they move closer to retirement. They worry about pain becoming worse as they prepare for the next stages in life, when they want to relax, do what they love doing, or take care of grandkids. Help yourself so that you can be pain-free and more active. Keep yourself healthy. Your loved ones would want that for you, too.

I'm afraid of the worst answer. Fearing the worst? The ideas and stories that fill our heads are the worst! Our brain is hard-wired that way because it's easier. It's easier to do nothing than it is to act. When you do act, that usually means researching on your computer. The stories we find online can also make us think the only answer is the worst answer. It doesn't have to be. If you look up Carpal Tunnel Syndrome, most of what you will read is how easy surgery is! You may read one sentence about going to physical or occupational therapy, but it doesn't go into depth about how a specialized therapist can help you avoid surgery. If I kept reading about the worst-case scenario, I guess I would be disheartened, too. I can tell you, as someone who specializes in hand and arm injuries, it is very possible to avoid that worst-case scenario. In a later chapter I will explain how you can take the first steps to get your questions answered, whether it be with another clinic or with us at Hands-on Therapy Services.

I want a fast, easy solution. I don't know of anything worth having that is fast or easy. Except McDonald's. Nothing that took years to create, like an imbalance in the body or a buildup of little injuries, takes one day or one visit to fix. Here at Hands-On Therapy Services we are dedicated to helping people over 40 because we know that, as we age, we accumulate little injuries that will require help at some point. Of course, we also help those with arm and hand injuries and surgeries, which can happen at any age.

As we mature, we tend to become more serious about our health. I've been working with a woman whom I met at a dinner. It took her six months before she decided to visit us because, honestly, she didn't have pain. Instead, she felt stiff all the time. She was planning on retiring soon and started to think about how she wanted to enjoy her time after years of hard work. She was worried about how working all those years had affected her neck, arms, and back. Now she visits us once a month for our wellness service in order to keep her body mobile, loose, and injury-free so that she can enjoy her retirement.

Everyone wants pain gone yesterday, but we are more realistic that all great things take effort. Pills and injections (cortisone or PRP) have a place in the world, but we know so many people who are looking for a more natural solution, without popping pills or getting injections. These things only mask the problem. It takes a little more effort to get to the root cause of your arm and hand issues and give you lasting results, so that you can arm yourself (pun intended!) with the knowledge of how you can help yourself in the future.

I don't have the time. If I could guarantee the results, would you make the time to get the help you need? Of course, yes! Sign me up! Unfortunately I can't guarantee results because there's me and there's you, and if you had surgery, there's the surgeon. There are too many factors that I can't control or have a direct impact on. Also, we don't know each other very well, but if I give you my time and attention and you give me yours, we can get to know each other better. That's how we can help you determine the best plan, because if you did put the time and effort in the right direction, you will get better results. It's like when you are driving from Miami to Orlando. You will get there in a timely manner if you planned your route and know exactly where you are going versus wandering around and guessing which direction to go. We want to work with people who are as committed as we are to achieving the best possible results. That's why we have free Discovery Visits, allowing people to come meet us in person before making any more commitments of time and money.

I have a client who is also a physical therapist. He cut his finger and had surgery. You might assume that, being a physical therapist, he would know what to do and would not need my help (in the next chapter I have a story about assumptions). I can tell you from my own experience that when I had knee surgery, other therapists assumed that I would be above getting help. I'm not. I'm just like you. I need help to be accountable, to be encouraged to do more for the best possible results, and to be led in the right direction. Because of my experience being discharged and told to do things on my own when I was barely able to walk without fear of falling, I do not and will not do that to others. The client was honest in telling me he wasn't taking the time to do the home program that we developed (life is crazy and very busy). However, he had just finished an incredible iron man race and crossed that finish line. I needed to remind him that he consistently trained, in key ways, to cross that finish line. How was his hand injury and surgery any different? Consistently coming to therapy, moving, and exercising were key ways to get the best results out of his hand surgery. We had to have that conversation. You would be willing to give yourself all the time you needed if you knew you could have the best results after any surgery or injury. You will make time for what is important to you. The key thing is seeing how important it is now and not waiting until your problem is worse or until you must think of the worst-case scenario.

It's too expensive. How expensive would surgery and the resulting therapy be? How expensive would it be if you could not work? How disruptive would that be to your work and family life if you suddenly had so much pain that you could not move your arm or required hand surgery?

I would urge you to hold off on making assumptions about cost. I may be so bold as to suggest that is fear stopping you from taking the necessary steps to know the truth. You might also be making assumptions about what you may or may not need. Therapy services do not need to be three times a week FOREVER! All our services are based on what you need, how quickly you may want to get better, and the time constraints that you have. Some surgeries are extremely time sensitive and require your therapy to be faster paced. But if you had hand and arm surgery, you would not be stuck over a decision to get started. You should be asking, who is best qualified to get me the best possible recovery? If you had kids or a parent who had surgery, you would not be asking, "Where can I go to get them the cheapest care?" You would be looking for a clinic that specializes in their injury and gives them the best possible chance for a full recovery.

Roadblocks

Those are a few of the mental roadblocks that my clients have told me about over and over through the years. It is human nature to have these mental roadblocks because they are easier than the UNKNOWN of "will therapy work for me?" This is normal. Everyone has these thoughts. What will you do about it, though?

Everyone who comes in and gets BETTER wishes that they had paid more attention and come in earlier, because they lost a lot of time. They lost time worrying, feeling uncomfortable, or being in pain. They lost time feeling limited and not doing what they wanted to do. They lost time because often waiting makes the problems worse.

Your body is the vehicle in life that takes you from place to place. You know that you need to take your vehicle in for tune-ups and oil changes and tire inspections for wear and tear. You do this so the daily drive for you and your family is safe and so you don't get stuck on the side of the road. Are you taking your body in for its proper tune-up? Where are you taking it? Are you taking your luxury vehicle to some general place or are you looking for the best mechanic in town to service your most prized vehicle?

Stop beating yourself up. It's okay. It's okay to have these thoughts and hesitations with any injury, but even more so with arm and hand problems. One of the main reasons people put it off for so long is because the problem hasn't yet stopped them. Your car is not yet broken down on the side of the road.

Let's be honest: it's about who you trust. Just like when finding a mechanic, you want to go to a place you trust and know won't take advantage of you. It's okay to be nice to yourself and give yourself a chance to feel great about your decision NOW. If you are stuck like we spoke about in Chapter One, and you want to avoid making these mental mistakes, keep reading to find out what steps you can take to improve how you are living.

How do you get unstuck?

So how do you get unstuck and not make the mistake of waiting with arm and hand problems?

How do you avoid those pitfalls and stories that you might tell yourself to delay getting help?

How do you avoid waiting for years with the potential of getting worse and missing out on living your best life?

If you are someone with hand and arms problems, this whole book is written just for you. If you know someone who is suffering, consider sharing this book with them. There are very few certified hand therapists – specialists in arm and hand problems – so I've compiled as much as I can to help you get unstuck. There are even fewer certified hand therapists in private practice who are solely devoted to helping you get unstuck from hand and arm problems.

Why continue being uncomfortable and in pain? It affects our moods, how we treat others, and how we allow others to treat us.

Imagine waking up comfortable in your body and getting ready without dreading painful hands. How nice might you be to your partner and kids because you feel good and not limited?

Imagine working and not feeling miserable because your elbows ache and you must constantly rub them, thinking that it's all that computer work that is making you miserable. How nice might it be to enjoy your day at work? That coworker might not be as annoying if you were feeling better.

Imagine working out or taking fitness classes and not having to hold back or miss out because you CAN do everything and are not limited by pain. How great would it be to hit your fitness goals, whether for strength or weight?

How wonderful would you feel on the inside and outside?

I hope you can relate to the tips, advice, and stories of others who have suffered with arm and hand problems. You can get more clarity about these problems, learn what you can do to get rid of them, and feel confident in your decisions about your health and well-being.

This book will tell you more about who we are at Hands-On Therapy Services and what we can do if you are having these arm and hand problems. Even if you don't choose us, you will be armed with some of the best knowledge we have to offer. You can know what questions to ask and how to find a place you can trust with your hands and arms.

Remember, taking no action at all when you have arm and hand problems is an action itself – with consequences. Feel great about your decision to read this book. Look for answers that satisfy you. And enjoy the stories.

Chapter 3

Why Suffer When You Don't Have to?

BEFORE I DIVE into why you may be suffering AND why you don't have to, I want to share a story. I'm not sure how funny it is without my face and body gestures and the changes in my voice, but you'll just have to imagine them.

I lovingly call it my "Prime Rib Story." Though it may seem like it has nothing to do with hand and arm therapy, it's a story that even my almost teenage son loves. It's a story about assumptions – how we all make assumptions and how assumptions can limit us. You decide and make choices based on them, so it's important not to let other people's assumptions limit you.

This happens to me just about every year during the holidays. At Christmas I host a large dinner for my family, and every year it gets bigger and bigger. If I do say so myself, I make an amazing prime rib that challenges all the fancy steakhouses. I dry-age it for at least three weeks and serve it with all the fixings and sides. My dad loves it, my father-in-law raves about it, and my husband can't wait each year for my prime rib.

I go into the supermarket and head for the meat department. I find this nice man and ask him, "I'm looking for the standing rib roast, the whole one. Can you please help me?"

He takes me over to the area, points to the packages that are there, and says, "Here are our standing rib roasts. They are on sale today."

"Great!" I reply. "I love a sale, but I want to buy the whole standing rib roast. Can you get that for me, please?"

He looks confused. "The whole standing rib?"

"Yes, I want the whole standing rib roast."

He holds his arms out to demonstrate how big the roast really is, and asks again: "The whole rib roast?"

"Yes." I say, holding my arms out to indicate that I want the largest one they have. "The whole rib roast. That's what I want."

Still looking confused, he goes to the back and brings it to the counter where I'm standing. He asks me, "Is this what you want, the whole rib roast?"

I chuckle and reply, "Yes, that's what I want. The whole standing rib roast. I need that, please."

So, he prints out the ticket and shows me the price tag. "You still want the whole rib roast?"

I say, laughing, "Yes, I still want the whole standing rib roast. It's Christmas, and I have a large party to host."

The man in the meat department made a lot of assumptions. He didn't ask me any questions to find out why I wanted a WHOLE standing rib roast. He couldn't understand why anyone would spend that much money. Most likely, not that many people come in to buy a whole rib roast. Maybe not that many people spend that much money on beef. Maybe no one who looks like me has ever asked for a WHOLE standing rib roast. He didn't know that my whole family looks forward to our Christmas dinner because of my devotion to creating an experience of culinary delight rivaling steakhouses. We get to be together in the comfort of our home, taking our time over dinner, with all the kids just running around. It's our tradition.

Who knows why he made those assumptions, but we ALL tend to make assumptions about situations that cross our paths. How is this related to hand therapy?

At Hands-On Therapy Services, we will not be making those assumptions. Most likely you are used to calling a health provider or therapy clinic where all they want to know is your name, date of birth, and insurance information. The only thing we want to know first is your name so that we may speak to you like a person. We will ask you questions about what is wrong, what you are looking for, what your goals are, and how fast or slow you want to take it. We want to get to know you. You may not be used to it because not many places do this. You might be the person asking, "Really? The whole rib roast?" Because it so rarely happens, right?

Here's WHY we do it. Therapy and your overall health and how your body works is NOT one-size-fits-all. It is not a pre-cut slab of standing rib roast. We will not make assumptions about what you want because we will ask all the questions necessary to make the best decision for YOU. Not for us. I know that is a foreign concept because you probably have not experienced this often – or ever. I know when I started my clinic five years ago and was the person answering the phone, our clients were surprised that they were talking to the specialist and had a chance to ask as many questions as they wanted. They were surprised that we were not making assumptions about them.

I want to encourage YOU not to make assumptions either. Here are some assumptions that we all tend to make, which leave us stuck having to suffer with indecision longer than necessary.

This is just what happens when people get old. Aging is a fact of life. No one can get around it. However, we don't have to live with the idea that age somehow makes us old. You DON'T get old and then get stiff. You get stiff, and then you FEEL old! I help people of all ages with arm and hand issues, but I have decided to focus on people age 40 and older because as we get older we NEED a little more help and accountability to stay healthier because it doesn't get easier. Young people in their 20s, 30s, 40s ALL tell me the SAME THING! "Oh, I have this because I am getting old." See? It has nothing to do with age. Not if everyone of all ages is telling me the same thing. Age is a mindset. Yes, we are prone to a few more problems. For example, tendinitis of the shoulder starts to surface in our 40s because we have put a lot of wear and tear on the most mobile and unstable joint in our body.

I was working with a client who is in her late 80s. Shirley lives by herself, drives where she wants to go, and still likes to play golf weekly. She had tripped on a door jam, falling and hurting her right arm. Of course, those who rushed to her aid only saw this older woman. When X-rays came back negative, they sent her home with a sling. Being as active as she was, she didn't stay in the sling very long, but she quickly realized that her arm was not getting completely better. She could use her arm but still had pain. Her doctors and friends told her it was due to age and that she should stop playing golf. It is unfortunate that doctors and friends, though well meaning, always tell you to "STOP doing" instead of "START doing."

When we met, she told me that it didn't make sense, because she was playing golf before the fall and was the same age. She figured there was something else still wrong with her shoulder. One day she went to an eye doctor who was understanding because he also loved to play golf. I truly believe he helped her find our therapy clinic, where we helped her get back to playing golf again. Shirley loved to tell us how she was the top golfer in her age bracket and how she won tournaments. Every time she came for her follow-up appointments, she was thrilled about how her golf score was getting better and how her golf friends praised her for how well she could swing her clubs at her age!

All I can say is that it's not the AGE thing! Call me a hopeless optimist, but I don't think it's about getting OLD and getting stiff but rather getting STIFF and feeling old!

We all have different types of bodies, and we all use them in different ways. Think about everything you used to do as a kid. Your experiences take a toll and shape your body differently. We tend to think that if we have pain today, it must be because we did something yesterday. And it may well be. But so many times, it's a cumulative effect of activities over time that really caused the problem.

I understand it's not so cut and dry when it comes to arm and hand issues. Where to go, who to see – so many options. We will address all of that in this book going forward, with chapter 11 all about how you can work with us. I do know that it is possible to live without aches and pains and worrying about the worst-case scenario, no matter the age. If anything, take care of it now, so you don't have to feel broken and need help in your 50s and 60s instead of being able to retire and enjoy life free of pain.

I need to go to the doctor first so that he/she can tell me for sure. We are conditioned from a young age always to go to the doctor when we have a question regarding our health. If that's what you need to feel good, then make a doctor's appointment and go. I am very pro-doctor. I have many in my family and have worked closely over my 20 years in practice with many different doctors whom I love and trust.

Some people ask me which specialist to go to, and I am happy to make a recommendation. At the end of the day, you know your body best and when you are honest about everything that is going on, it makes recommending which specialist easier. For example, when you describe certain symptoms and report that you have pain at different joints in many different parts of your body, and you are a certain age, a rheumatologist is a great specialist to see. Or if you say that you have numbness or nerve issues, a neurologist is the specialist you might need.

My concern with going to the doctor first or ONLY is that when the problem is not severe, you delay and put off going to the doctor, which delays you even longer from getting the help you need. If that is what you are telling yourself before you seek help from therapy, the problem will only get worse.

My other concern is that not all doctors recommend therapy services first – or ever! They may recommend pills or recommend injections. Not because they don't want to help. It's because not all doctors truly know what we can do as therapists, and they don't always know the best places to send you.

My own mother went to her primary care doctor about her shoulder pain because she grew up in a time when there was an inherent trust of what the doctors tell you, even though I was already helping her to get rid of the pain. I asked her why she felt a need to go even as she was getting better, and she said "because I wanted to know for sure." Of course, I told her exactly what was going to happen. After she came back, she said, "Yup, he offered me pills for the pain and an injection." She declined only because I cautioned her about it, knowing my mother doesn't like to take pills and did not want an injection. He sent her to therapy only when she asked. He also sent her to a place where he is contracted to send her, leaving her with no choices. They barely touched her, treating her alongside four to five other patients. It's a no wonder she was not getting better. She only told me about all of this after I started working with her.

If you need to go to the doctor for peace of mind, I won't try stop you. You don't have to wait, however. You can access therapy without a prescription. We can help you get more clarity and, if you need to go to a doctor, we can recommend which specialist may help you best. Getting started, especially with therapy services, is always the best path so you don't keep delaying for another day. It's a service I am proud to offer to you. Speak to a specialist at our clinic first (https://www.handsots.com/talk-to-the-therapist/), so that we can discuss how to help you before booking any paid appointments.

I need to have a test to know for sure. You want to "see" what that problem could be because you want definite answers. There is a place for them. For example, if you fell and got injured, or if you have been getting help from other professionals but you don't feel better. Let me break it down because, as useful as they are, these tests are over used and often do not help you get any closer to solving your problem.

1. X-ray – It gives you a picture of what's going on with your bones at the one area that you have pain. Is your joint sitting in the right place? Is your bone broken? It does not tell you why you have pain. It doesn't tell you the root cause of the pain either.
2. MRI – It gives you a picture of the surrounding soft tissues, like ligaments, tendons, and bones. MRIs are great if you suspect a ligament or tendon is torn. It's also great if you are considering surgery because it is ordered to see if your surgery can be justified for insurance coverage.
3. Nerve conduction test – It gives you insight into how much your nerve, as well as which nerve, is compressed. This also determines if you qualify for surgery.

After the test, however, what were you hoping it would tell you? Tests don't tell you anything that you don't already know. They only confirm that you have a problem. It does not fix your pain or problems. You already know where you hurt. You already know that you are having difficulty reaching behind to put on your bra, or difficulty lifting weights, or lifting your kids to play with them, or difficulty waking up with numbness and stiffness. You already feel those problems. The tests qualify you for surgery.

This happened to a physical therapy friend of mine:

A potential client of his said, "I'm really curious to try therapy with you."

My therapist friend said, "I can help you know with this technique that has helped others just like you."

She said, "No thanks. I have an MRI next week, and I don't want to mess that up."

The therapist said, "You are worried I might make you feel better?'

"Well, kind of. I want to be hurting when I have the test," she responded.

YES, I promise this happened. This happened with a client of mine as well! She came to talk to us about her carpal tunnel but didn't want to get started with therapy because she didn't want to mess up the nerve conduction test. She didn't want to have surgery. She was adamant about not having surgery because then she wouldn't be able to take care of her grandkids. But it was hurting her a lot when she did take care of them throughout the week. It took her two months before she had anything tested. She made her appointment to come in once they recommended surgery.

She waited 15 years because she had the nerve conduction test years before but didn't qualify for surgery. She lived with the problem until it became a problem of her hands, elbows, and shoulders. You don't have to be stuck waiting around for doctor's appointments and tests to get the help you need and want. Get the tests if that is the only way to get peace of mind, but then get the actual help to get rid of the pain and problems before they get worse.

I went somewhere, and it didn't really help. Had a bad experience? OR a not-so-great one? We have all been to a doctor. It's not always pleasant. It may not be "bad," but not one that we are rushing out to go to. The waiting – and the waiting – and only to get two minutes with the doctor. Maybe five minutes if you are lucky. If you are going because you have a bad cold and want some meds, the doctor not spending time with you is not a problem, because in those two minutes they give you a prescription medication that can get to the root cause of your infection. When you have pain and need help, that's different. Offering pain medications or injections doesn't give you all the answers that you need, nor do they get to the root cause of the problem. You need more.

Going to a physical/occupational therapist is no different. Have you been to a clinic where the staff barely look up from what they are doing to have a conversation with you? Have you been to a place where you sit with four to five other people waiting in line for time and attention, not getting the results that you want? If you leave those places lacking the urge to go back, no wonder it didn't help.

Don't you want to come into a pleasant environment where people seem to care about how you are feeling? Don't you want to find a place that will give you **all the time and attention that you want** and will talk to you about how they can solve your problem and develop an action plan of what that can look like? It may sound crazy, but places like this exist! Hands-On Therapy Services is one of those places. And if you are not in Miami to experience it, then you should be. But seriously, it is possible for you to find clinics like us in other parts of the country too.

I recently helped a young woman with elbow problems. I was just blown away at how proactive she was. She had a persistent, achy pain that would occur whenever she played her musical instrument. She tried therapy somewhere else and didn't have a bad experience with it. She said the therapist was perfectly nice but didn't pay attention to what she needed. It didn't get rid of the problem completely. She worried because she values how much she uses her arms for her work. If she couldn't work, it wasn't just money but her whole career. The more she played, the more the pain came back. I loved that she kept looking for a different solution and found us online. From our website she was able to request to speak with the specialist (https://www.handsots.com/talk-to-the-therapist/) to get a better understanding of how we could help. Then we invited her for a free Discovery Visit before booking any paid sessions.

Having already gone somewhere else and tried other things, she saved us time so that we could work that much better to find a solution to her problem. That gave us fast results from day one. We were able to dig in based on what she was doing before, what worked, and what didn't to create a new plan of action for her. We created a plan that she can continue on her own, once we were able to solve the problem. So if you have tried other therapy clinics that didn't solve your problem completely, it's still possible. It's about finding a place that will ask you the right questions to find the best solution for you.

I don't know who to trust. – That's an easy one! AND hard one at the same time. Go to as many people as you need to get answers! Why only go to Google for answers? Why only go to one doctor for suggestions? Sometimes it takes more than one specialist. How many specialists do you talk to when consulting for a boob job or when having heart surgery? If someone does not make you feel confident and COMFORTABLE about their services, it's possible that you can find someone else. You know your body better than anyone else. Find someone who specializes in your problem and gives you the time and attention that you want.

One of our clients had gone to three or four different therapy clinics before coming to ours. He was not happy with the overall experience and lack of results after a wrist surgery, so before taking him on as a client we gave him the time and attention to answer his questions and make him comfortable with how we do business. He stayed and came back because of the experience we were able provide and results we were able to deliver. It was possible that he would need to have a second surgery if he did not improve, so he needed to feel confident about his decision. I encouraged him to seek as many opinions as he felt comfortable with. In the end, he went to two other orthopedics that were recommended by us, and he settled on the one that made him feel most comfortable. He was happy with how we treated him and with the results – without another surgery. Most importantly, he did enough research to make himself confident and comfortable. I know it is hard to find someone you can trust, in all aspects of life, not just in the health world. You'll feel good when you can trust a person or a place to give you solid advice.

I was told I'm supposed to do it on my own. I can't even begin to tell you how many times I have heard this coming from our clients who have been elsewhere. Whether you are avoiding surgery or had surgery, some people (friend, doctors, insurance, other therapists) will tell you that you need to continue on your own in order to get to 100%. I can tell you with all of my being that there is so much potential for you to get there but we can't always do it on our own. Most of us, and I say us because I include myself in this, need help and accountability. Most people, especially after surgery, think, "I am so much better because I have full motion and am able to do so much more on my own now." You ARE better, and you CAN do more on your own. Don't assume, however, that you can't get a little extra help when you need it to get where you can feel loose, strong, and great. It takes time and attention to get to 100% recovery.

After my own knee surgery many years ago, the physical therapist discharged me (to my surprise) and gave me a packet of exercises that she told me to do. She assumed that I would be able to do them on my own. I'll be honest, life was busy, and I didn't keep it up. I recently helped a friend who came in from out of town who had a similar story with her feet surgery issues. Her therapist had discharged her with a packet of exercises and told her she could do her home program on her own. She was able to walk without pain. She came for our wellness service and told me that two years after her surgery her feet were still tight,she could not wear certain shoes, and she could not walk as far and as fast as she would like. Other issues were starting to surface. I was able to advise her on what to look for and which questions to ask when she sought help near her home.

All the time we have clients who, after arm and hand surgery (and leg and feet surgery), need reminders of what they need to do, even coming in for "tune-up" sessions. In the next few chapters, you will read about their stories. One who had a distal radius fracture went off to school and had to do his stretches and exercises on his own but school was so busy! So when he came home for break, he came in for a tune-up session. Another came for shoulder stretches and an update on what exercises were still important. Lots of people assume that because of surgery they will never be the same again. They don't give themselves the opportunity to be the same when others assume that they don't need help again and that they can do it ALL on their own. We all need help at different points. Don't cheat yourself from making a 100% recovery that will let you do what you want to be able to do without pain because someone else made assumptions about you.

Assumptions

What other assumptions are you making that are holding you back? You don't have to feel old because of a number. You don't have to wait for doctors or expensive tests that only point you toward surgery. You don't have to give up because one place or one person told to you give up. You don't have to do it all on your own. Sometimes, it's their assumptions about you that are holding you back. Sometimes, it's your assumptions about what is possible that are holding you back. You don't have to keep suffering or worrying.

The next few chapters are about the arm and hand problems that we have been helping people overcome for more than 20 years. There are plenty of stories of the wonderful people with whom we have crossed paths, and there are tips and advice that you can start using to get yourself unstuck. Know that you don't have to keep waiting, wondering, and suffering.

Chapter 4

On The One Hand

Carpal Tunnel Syndrome

I COULD PROBABLY TALK about hands ALL DAY LONG! I know from asking people with different injuries that they think their legs and walking are important. And they ARE important. But without hands, you can't manipulate the things in your environment, and you lose a different type of independence. After working with hundreds of people over the last 20 years, I know that people don't fully appreciate their hands until there is an injury. Then they realize how much they need their hands for everything that they do. It's as simple as pressing a button and as intimate as wiping your ass (I mean, seriously, have you ever had to wipe with your non-dominant hand?!).

Our hands are one of the most complex body parts. Not only do our hands help to pick up a sandwich or glass of water, but they also allow us to move small objects such as coins within our fingers. The nerves feed our brains with information on everything we feel, such as whether something is hot or cold. Our fingertips let us know when something feels smooth or when something feels prickly. Without sensation, we would drop things constantly and would have to use our eyes to give our brain information on what we hold. We need to know we are putting the right amount of pressure whether we are pressing down to write or cradling a ripe piece of fruit. We need our hands not only to close into a fist but also to open our fingers wide. We need to be able to feel all of what we are doing and touching. Because of all that our hands can do, our hand functions take up a large space in our brain.

Hand injuries are among the most complex of all injuries. They can also be among the most devastating, especially if the injury is to your dominant hand (or both hands). Hand problems and injuries can be broken into three different parts. In this chapter, I will explain the most common hand injuries and how you can take steps to avoid the worst case of pills, injections and surgery.

- Wrist – Carpal tunnel, De Quervain's tendinitis, wrist tendinitis, sprains
- Hand – Trigger fingers or thumbs
- Fingers – Arthritis, sprains, and dislocations of the finger, finger jam types of injuries

Injuries to the wrist can include things like sprains, wrist tendinitis, De Quervain's tendinitis, and carpal tunnel syndrome. Yes! Carpal tunnel syndrome is a wrist problem even though if you have carpal tunnel issues, you will feel the problems in your hands and tips of your fingers.

What is Carpal Tunnel Syndrome?

Carpal tunnel syndrome is when the median nerve gets compressed or essentially choked at the wrist area. The carpal tunnel area is right at the middle base of the wrist. It's full of bones and tendons, with the nerve in the middle. The median nerve can be compressed because of what we do all day. When the muscles become tight, small amounts of swelling and scarring in that area build up over time, causing more pressure to build up, slowly but surely compressing the nerve. The median nerve starts from the neck and travels down through the arm and into the wrist. All along the way, there are key areas that can also get compressed, such as the neck or shoulder area. Most of the time those areas are overlooked.

What happens when you THINK you might have carpal tunnel?

Due to the compression, you may have some of these common symptoms:

- Night pain that wakes you up and makes you want to shake out your hands
- Numbness on the tips of the thumb, index finger, middle finger, and sometimes, when it's bad, half of the ring finger
- Pins and needles or a tingling sensation
- Achiness during the day
- Feeling uncomfortable
- Feeling clumsy
- Hands feeling weak
- Painful hands
- Atrophy, when the muscle is wasted away, such that you can see hollowness in certain parts of your hand

Carpal Tunnel Syndrome is by far the most talked about diagnosis of the hand. Most people have had it or have heard about it from friends or family members who have had it. If you tell someone that your hand hurts and you feel numbness, I am 99% sure they will say you probably have carpal tunnel. I can't really do that experiment because as soon as I tell someone that I am a hand specialist, THEY are the ones who tell me about carpal tunnel. Some people do research online and learn what they can do on their own to get better. If they are not sure, and it's lasting for weeks or months, they usually will consider going to a doctor first. But which doctor should they go to for help? That alone makes them think, "Ugh, do I really want to spend my time waiting there? What will they actually do for me?"

Most of the time you might even wait longer for help because it's not stopping you from doing anything, you don't want to wait at the doctors office, and you don't know there is an option to go directly to get help from a specialized hand therapist.

If you do make it to a doctor's appointment, they will likely confirm what you already suspected and issue you a prefabricated splint, one that is one-size-fits-all (or as I say, one-size-fits-none, although some of them are actually a pretty good fit when it's for carpal tunnel). They will tell you to wear it, prescribe some pills for inflammation, and then tell you to come back in four to six weeks. But you don't necessarily want to wear that splint. And when and for how long do you wear it? And do you REALLY want to go back after waiting weeks for an appointment only to get two minutes with the doctor if you're lucky?

Another option that some doctors will offer is an injection. They may just tell you to wait until the pain gets worse so that you can have surgery, because it's an easy surgery to get rid of the carpal tunnel. Does this process sound familiar to you? I've heard this often from those I have helped. Most of them tell me THIS IS THE WHOLE REASON why they end up waiting SO LONG before getting any kind of help. One woman who called us said she agreed to an injection, which helped her numbness for a few days, but then her hand started to hurt more, all the way up her arm. Another woman told me her doctor said, "Oh, you will need surgery for that," so she ended up waiting 15 years – FIFTEEN YEARS! – to do anything about it.

All of this can leave you feeling frustrated, annoyed and, most of all, drive you crazy! The pain may not STOP you from getting things done, but it can surely slow you down. I think that is one of the MAIN reasons people mistakenly let it go for way too long. There is NOTHING wrong with what the doctors are offering you. I don't want you to think that I am bad-mouthing doctors. So many of them are great, and I personally work very closely with many doctors in the Miami and Fort Lauderdale area. But if you go to ask them, they will give you THEIR best answers. There is nothing wrong with injections and surgery. There is a place for them in this world! If YOU don't want that and are trying to avoid medications, injections and surgery, doctors are NOT the first line of defense to get you the help you need. The right Occupational/Physical Therapists that specialize in hand problems are the most natural solution. Medications and injections can have side effects. Surgery is easy for surgeons because it literally takes them FIVE MINUTES to complete the procedure. It takes longer to prep you than it does to have the surgery. Consider other types of hand surgeries and carpal tunnel release is relatively easy. But it will take YOU a minimum of three to six months for a full recovery. So, no, surgery is not easy for you. Would you be interested in NOT having to take pills or injections and AVOIDING surgery?

Did you know that women are THREE TIMES MORE LIKELY than men to have Carpal Tunnel Syndrome? You may have been told by a doctor, a friend, or a family member that you have Carpal Tunnel Syndrome, and you may have researched it on your own, coming to the same conclusion. The first thing they often tell you is to put on a brace and to "rest" your hands or even "stop" whatever you are doing. Most of the time it's paired with "take some pills" and "lets wait to see if it gets worse." When it is bad enough, doctors will recommend a nerve conduction test. Then they'll recommend an injection or, worse, surgery.

Most of the time healthcare providers are treating this problem generically. They only look at your wrist, keep you in a brace, and give you stretches and exercises that can even make the carpal tunnel worse. Truth is, it's standard practice to have you stop doing "that thing" that they think you are doing. Remember that most people tell you to "STOP doing" instead of "START doing." The last thing you want to do is slow down or stop, because as a busy person with a career and family there is no choice but to continue going full speed ahead.

I've talked to career people who sit at a desk on the computer all day or just have one of those jobs that are active and require them to use their hands. As I was getting ready to do some writing on the subject of carpal tunnel, a retired nurse, Rachal, happened to come in and ask us about the carpal tunnel nerve conduction test that her doctor had ordered. Turns out, as we were talking and getting to know each other, she had been suffering for at least 15 YEARS! She has been retired for the past year, and her hands are getting better. Yet since she started to care for her grandkids, her hands have started hurting again. She's been feeling tight, weak, and getting the pins and needles sensation more and more. It's driving her CRAZY. It also makes her feel very restricted in what she can do in her everyday life and retirement. But as Rachal said, she was diagnosed with Carpal Tunnel Syndrome years ago. They recommended surgery for her, but she didn't know that occupational/hand therapy could help. She didn't want surgery because it would have stopped her from working, but now that she is retired, she is taking care of her grandkids, and her hands are getting worse. Imagine! She has been suffering with this for AT LEAST 15 YEARS! I hear stories just like hers all the time. You don't have to suffer like that.

Pregnant women – and moms, too – suffer quite a lot when it comes to Carpal Tunnel Syndrome. If you are pregnant, your chance of having gestational carpal tunnel skyrockets! That can be due to weight gain and fluid retention all over your body, but especially in your hands and wrist area, and especially during the second and third trimester as your baby grows! It's exciting that the baby is getting better and bigger! But as one mom-to-be told me, "that pain and numbness is pretty restrictive." There's not a lot of space there for anything extra. When there's more fluid, it chokes that median nerve, which is why you get the night pain and numbness. In general, it will go away after the baby is born.

Occasionally carpal tunnel syndrome does not go away after having the baby. A friend of mine developed Carpal Tunnel Syndrome toward the end of her pregnancy, and she didn't gain that much weight. Even so, there was a certain amount of water retention. After having the baby, her discomfort got better but the numbness got worse again when the baby was 3 months old. It drove her CRAZY! If you are breastfeeding, your body is still having raging hormones. Your body went through a major change by carrying another human being. Therefore, it takes some time to get over those changes. Outside of that, you get even BUSIER taking care of your family and all the things that it entails. That means you are using your hands even more. Those babies don't get any lighter, either. Getting the help you need to end your carpal tunnel aches and numbness is key to making sure it doesn't get so bad that you must consider more invasive procedures like injections and surgery. Those can slow you down even MORE!

Carpal tunnel can also happen as a result of an accident, such as a fall on your arm, or of surgery for a fracture of the wrist or elbow. People may experience lots of swelling, which takes a long time to get rid of, or they may become stiff in certain areas, compressing the carpal tunnel nerve. Recently, we were helping someone after biceps tendon repair. He kept feeling numbness that wouldn't ease up in his arm and fingers. The difficult part was that his elbow was doing well in terms of the recovery, but his wrist was tight! It had been tight from the beginning, when he was swollen all the way down to his arm and hands. With all that swelling and tightness from the biceps/elbow injury, he now had persistent numbness that wasn't going away. In his normal day-to-day activities before the surgery to fix the tendon, he had never experienced numbness like this. Developing carpal tunnel after surgery or a fall is much different from a slow onset of Carpal Tunnel Syndrome.

What IS easy for you to do is look for a certified hand therapist/occupational therapist who can help you with what YOU can do. This kind of therapist can look at the whole picture to find the root cause of the problem and determine where the compression is along the median nerve. We work with clients who are serious about getting to the root cause of their carpal tunnel and eliminating it in the most natural way.

Want to avoid all of this and get the help you need? Want to avoid pills, injections and surgery? Here are my FIVE MAIN TIPS to start getting rid of Carpal Tunnel Syndrome WITHOUT surgery!

1. **Wearing a wrist support splint.** ONLY at night! Do it every night for at least a month, even when you think you are feeling better. You must be consistent. Trying a pre-fabricated one from the drug store is easy. There's a small metal bar in the middle that positions your wrist a little back. It's called wrist extension. The key is to bend the bar until it is straight, so that it holds your wrist completely STRAIGHT. That will help relieve any pressure in that area for more blood flow during the night. Wearing a splint is just the start and should be used in conjunction with other treatment methods. Some people think this is the end-all be-all and use it for YEARS without real relief from carpal tunnel. They also start using it during the day as well, which usually develops a totally different problem. I recommend weaning from the splint after two to three months of night use, depending on the severity and whether the problem is truly at the wrist level.

Stretch your fingers and wrist wide open and back. We use our hands a lot, especially for gripping and squeezing. When they start hurting or feeling weak, we adjust the ways we use them, causing more of an imbalance. It's great to stretch the fingers open and the wrist back, doing a composite stretch to alleviate the tension at that carpal tunnel area. I recommend to start with wrist and hand stretches, but there are a variety of shoulder, neck, and nerve stretches that can also help. Not sure how to do it? There are many different ways, and we have sample videos on our Youtube channel. You can also request them by visiting our website (www.handsots.com). Subscribe to our YouTube channel to stay up to date with any new releases on videos.

2. **STOP squeezing a ball!** Don't constantly squeeze your hands. It's the worst thing you can do. I know, even the doctors and friends tell you to squeeze a ball when you tell them that your hands feel very weak. It's not because you are "weak," it's because the nerve is being choked and slowing down the messages to your muscles. To keep squeezing the ball or constantly making a fist is to continue choking that median nerve even more. I guarantee you are doing it more than you think, and this may be the one thing that is making you feel worse.

3. **Use heat on your hands and wrist area.** It will help make your hands feel better and relieve the achiness. This tip does NOT get to the root cause, but it makes it more bearable until you decide to get the help you need to get rid of it completely. Why heat instead of ice? Since this is a nerve problem, heat can help. Ice has been shown to be more effective when you've just had an injury, and I have found that muscles respond to and like the cold when they are feeling tight and sore. Nerves like heat better than they do the cold.

4. **My final tip: Don't wait; get the help you need from a certified hand therapist.** Get the relief you need before it gets WORSE. I've had people wait YEARS, and I mean YEARS, without the help they need. I was in a Facebook group of moms. The ladies there were chatting about all the hand pain, tingling, numbness they were STRUGGLING with. Not knowing where to go, worried about what it was. Could it get worse? What it would mean to their lives if their hand got worse. Injections and surgery scared them. They didn't want to take pills. But they waited and suffered for YEARS. One mom would tell another, "Oh no, don't do therapy or go to the doctor. All you have to do is 'this' and it will get better." But in the same post they would say that the pain "would come and go" and that they still have to be "careful" about doing this one thing or not doing this one thing. Other moms would read that and think,

39

"Oh well, if they are suffering and not getting better, then maybe I won't get better either." Another story is, "Oh, I just waited, and it totally went away for me although I didn't do anything." Not everyone gets better. Most people need help. More than 8 million people are affected by Carpal Tunnel Syndrome. It is THE SECOND MOST COMMON musculoskeletal surgery performed each year. That's a lot of surgeries for something that can be prevented from getting worse.

My recommendation for carpal tunnel syndrome is to try the suggestions above. If you truly are trying and still suffering for months, there is something that can be done about carpal tunnel. You also don't have to play the waiting game of it coming and going. Find the root cause of why you are having those symptoms, learn what you can do to get rid of it for good, and also be armed with the skills to know what to do if it were to come back. It doesn't have to be tons of therapy sessions either, like you might have if you had surgery. Consider this: if you are suffering, what would it be worth to get a full night's rest, like when you were younger and didn't have to wear those braces on your hands? What is it worth to have peace of mind, knowing you can get help?

10 Reasons Why Waiting Is WORSE

1. Numbness and tingles will get worse
2. You can't sleep because the night pain keeps waking you up, and now you are struggling during the day
3. The pain slows you down (imagine what you could do if you didn't have numbness and pain)
4. You start realizing how much you compensate, while other parts of your arm start to develop other problems (trust me when I say that just about everyone I help – after waiting for years – has other elbow, hand, or shoulder issues)
5. You have weakness of the hand and arm

6. You worry about what else can happen
7. Takes longer to treat and is more difficult to get a full recovery
8. You experience atrophy, the slow choking of the nerve that starts to kill the muscle, which is not reversible.
9. You have to take pills or use the splint longer than you would like
10. You must have surgery, which has a lengthy recovery

Did you know that once the nerve has been compressed and deprived of oxygen, there's a certain amount of nerve death that occurs? Once that happens, it can be nearly impossible to get it back. Once that happens, numbness starts to stick around, and it can get worse and worse. Even if you have surgery, you may not get all that numbness to go away. This is what can happen if you WAIT. Muscle death. The fancy word for it is atrophy. That's when the nerve is compressed so long that it no longer can send signals to activate the muscle. Even with surgery the amount of atrophy doesn't fully recover. These are some of the main reasons why it's so important NOT TO WAIT to help your hands. Take care of them before the pain, numbness and weakness set in and you can't change it.

At Hands-On Therapy Services, we are the **TOP private hand therapy center in the Miami area,** helping people like you who are suffering from carpal tunnel hand pain and numbness get the advice and help you need to make the best decision about your quality of life. We do a thorough exam to check all areas of the median nerve path to find out where it is being compressed. That allows us to get to the root cause of the pain and numbness. There's no need to continue suffering from night pain that wakes you up or the morning feeling of pins and needles in your hands. There's no need to keep waiting until the pain is so bad and the numbness and weakness become permanent. There are ways to avoid surgery and long-term suffering. It is possible for you to get the help you need.

Is It Really Necessary?

YES! You REALLY do need help.

We look at every part of the neck, shoulders, elbow, wrist, and hand. We take ALL of that into account, and we do hands-on testing in the clinic to see where you might be stuck, where your nerve is tight, and where it could be choked. We take a thorough look at our arms and hands AND ask key questions to find the root cause of what is going on – how you use them, how you sleep, anything that can help you get rid of carpal tunnel once and for all without surgery. We want to get you "Started" doing what you want, not "Stop" you.

If you want, you can go to the doctor. I say this because a lot of people tell me they want to only to come back saying, "Yeah, it was a waste of time." But listen, we ALL grew up thinking that if something is wrong, go to the doctor. If you are sick, go to the doctor. If you are in pain, go to the doctor. I grew up like that, too, so I totally get it! I tell my clients to go to the doctor if that's what gives them peace of mind. But this will most likely happen: you start to tell the doctor what's wrong, and without touching you or anything, they will say, "Sounds like you have carpal tunnel." They will prescribe a splint to wear, pills to take, and recommend that you do a nerve conduction test. If you go to a hand doctor, they may do a little bit more in the office. Most nerve conduction tests are done at a neurologist's office or at a testing facility, which is just MORE TIME. I understand the lure of the nerve conduction test because everyone thinks it will give them a clear, written-down, black-and-white picture of "something" that is wrong in the carpal tunnel. However, it only tests for one part of the nerve, and depending on the results, you either are recommended for injection or surgery.

The surgeon will tell to you how easy the surgery is. I've been there when they speak about it. I've been in surgery with some of the top hand surgeons. It's an EASY surgical procedure – for THEM. They are in and out in five minutes. But YOUR recovery time is not five minutes NOR is it easy! It can take months to recover. We helped one woman, Maria, who had surgery on her right hand because it was the worst, and she had planned to go back in a month to have surgery on the left hand. She didn't realize how stiff and painful it would be because the doctor told her it was a simple surgery, that she could start moving right away, and that she could return to work. But it was NOT EASY for her. Her hand was so painful and so stiff after the surgery that she was taking a lot of pain medications. She didn't know what she was going to do because she needed to have surgery on her other hand. Maria started coming to us for treatments for right surgical hand, and we were able to help her with BOTH hands. She canceled the surgery to the left hand. She was able to return to working without pain in her hands, and she slept through the night. Maria was able to spend time with her family without feeling annoyed and frustrated by her hands.

Rarely will doctors recommend hand therapy, even though hand therapy is the most natural, conservative method of eliminating numbness and pain by getting to the root cause of carpal tunnel. Even if doctors DO recommend hand therapy, a lot of people tell me they end up not going because they are not sure how therapy can help or where they should go.

PLEASE don't wait 15 or 20 or 25 years, when it's so bad that even surgery will not turn back the clock, to let yourself live a more comfortable, enjoyable life.

We are not looking to help everyone. We are looking to help people who are serious about getting the help they need to AVOID surgery. As a certified hand therapist for nearly 20 years, I know how people are told to wear a splint, stretch at home – or worse, squeeze a ball – and wait until the pain is bad enough that the insurance company will approve surgery. Recover faster and get help from someone who values your TIME and provides you with the expert help you need, using specific testing and a proven program to get to the root cause of our hand pain and numbness, and then helping you fix it and empowering you to fix it on your own if the symptoms ever reappear.

We are looking to help YOU

- Who are suffering from night pain and can't get a full night of sleep
- Who are having numbness and tingling that is driving you crazy
- Who are feeling frustrated
- Who are feeling worried
- Who want to have a better quality of life without slowing yourself down
- Who have tried the DIY thing without getting the results you hoped for
- Who want to AVOID surgery

If you value your health and wellbeing, I hope you will consider getting help for your carpal tunnel. Don't put it off any longer. Later in this book, I will help you figure which is the best way to get started with us OR with someone else outside the Miami area.

Chapter 5

On The Other Hand

De Quervain's Tendinitis, and
Thumb & Finger Injuries

YOU KEEP HEARING this word "tendinitis," and it seems like it's everywhere and can happen anywhere in the body. That is true, but there are areas that are more prone to tendinitis. The wrist area is small, full of tight areas, and jam-packed with tendons. Tendinitis can happen on the thumb side (radial side) or the pinky side (ulnar side) of your wrist.

De Quervain's is also known as radial styloid tenosynovitis. It is usually pain around the thumb/wrist area, noticed when you grab something like a jug of milk or turn a door knob. De Quervain's is the inflammation of the tendons that open the thumb (extensor pollicis brevis and the abductor pollicis longus) in the area near the wrist. A thin tissue (the sheath) that holds the tendons in place can get thick and make it difficult for the tendon to glide. Every person's anatomy is different in that area, making it hard to know why it happens in some people and not in others.

Repetition of motions – such as heavy gripping with a twisting of the wrist while opening jars, grabbing thick charts, cutting with scissors, or holding forceps – are factors that can cause pain at the thumb/wrist area. A fall on an outstretched hand or sudden wrenching of the hand during a fight can also cause pain at the thumb/wrist area. De Quervain's tendinitis also tends to occur more among females than males, especially between the ages of 35 to 55. Not to say you cannot have it otherwise, but it's more common during these ages. In my professional experience, I have treated many more women than men. Usually with men there's an acute trauma that has caused it. Whereas, in women that I have treated, it is due to the repetitive nature of various tasks. Occasionally, it can arise during or after pregnancy.

So now you have pain. Perhaps you know how you got it or at least what it is. What can you do about it? How can you reduce the irritation and pain? It's hard because we need our hands for everything. At first, it doesn't always hurt. Only when you do that gripping, twisting motion. Then it will start to hurt more and more without doing anything. Please don't let it get to that point, because by then, it's much harder to get rid of it.

Here are a few tried and true tips that I give to my clients with De Quervain's Tendinitis.

- Use a well-fitted "thumb spica" splint during the day, especially when doing heavy activity. Use it for several weeks while you help to reduce the pain. Take it off at different times of the day and move your hand and wrist in a pain-free way
- Temporarily reduce the motion that irritates the tendon the most, which is heavy gripping while twisting at the wrist. It's not forever, only while you are working to reduce the inflammation, because the whole point is to get back to doing everything without limits.
- Massage the area, especially if it is swollen.
- Give it an ice massage. Get a cube of ice or a frozen cup and directly massage the area for 3-5 minutes.

If you go to the doctor, many will issue you a prefabricated thumb spica splint or direct you to buy one. Sometimes that's great, and it's certainly the cheapest option. But pay attention to how it fits your hand. The tip of your thumb should be sticking out, and you should be able to bend the little knuckle of the thumb all the way down and all the way up. The splint should only stop you from moving your wrist and part of your thumb. I know it's cheaper than a custom-fitted orthosis (splint), and that's why most people get the prefabricated ones from the drug store, but it may not always be the best fitting. When it is not fitting well, it will cause you MORE pain and stiffness! To get a well-fitted splint, visit us at Hands-On Therapy Services, where we will make you a custom-fitted splint. There is some research that says if your wrist is placed slightly in ulnar deviation (angled a little to the side of the pinky) it can be even more helpful. However, that's not possible with a splint that you buy at the store.

Besides the splinting, which is forcing you to rest that hand and wrist to let the swelling go down, make sure you remove the splint at times and gently move your thumb and wrist in a pain-free way so that you do not get stiff. Using something like that is great for reducing the pain, but being stuck in a splint is usually what makes people with De Quervain's even worse over time. You can also massage the area to help get rid of any swelling that is stuck there and free any scar tissue that is hardening up that area. I am a huge proponent of icing to reduce the pain and swelling. I also like to use Kinesio taping to help with the pain without having to use the splint. It allows you to use your hand with ease. Studies show, however, that in the most painful stages, splinting does help. Occupational therapy/hand therapy can be a big help not only to get rid of the pain in a natural way but also get to the root cause of the problem and prevent it from coming back. If you are not sure how much to move or what exactly you need to do, call us or visit our website and request to speak to our specialists (www.handsots.com).

Some people get injections at the doctor's suggestion. Others would rather avoid all medications, especially cortisone injections. Cortisone injections can be effective at getting rid of the pain faster, but not beyond two injections. If you are looking simply to get rid of it faster, you can talk to your doctor to determine if that is the right option for you. Most of the time, injections in this area do help with the pain when you have a bad case, but you may have a risk of the pain returning since you did not fix the root cause. One of the things to consider is how fast the symptoms return.

Surgery is considered only if you have tried all the conservative methods and nothing has worked at stopping the pain and allowing you to be fully functional in all your activities. It is usually a persistent interference with the quality of living and working that gets people to the point where they are ready for surgery. After surgery, you will need some occupational therapy/certified hand therapy to help you with your pain, scarring, and motion.

If you are looking to avoid the pain getting worse, stop the pain from slowing you down and making you feel like there are certain things you cannot do, and get the most natural treatment, give occupational therapy/hand therapy with Hands On Therapy Services a try sooner rather than later.

Other kinds of tendinitis

Tendinitis pain on the ulnar side of the wrist is less common and less known than De Quervain's. If you are having pain at your wrist on the pinky side, it may be what is called an ECU or FCU tendinitis, which means it's painful to a very specific tendon called the extensor carpi ulnaris or the flexor carpi ulnaris. The muscles start at the elbow and end on the pinky side of your wrist, but they can become sore and painful over time. Ulnar-sided pain can occur like all other types of tendinitis – sore and achy, sometimes feeling tight or sharp, then it dissipates. I generally don't recommend using a splint for these types of tendinitis. Using braces to stop movement tends to make you stiff and weak and can cause other compensatory bad habits that are hard to stop. Untreated, these types of tendinitis usually develop into tennis elbow or golfer's elbow (see Elbow chapter) or the other way around.

The right therapy program is the best chance to get rid of the wrist pain. Injections and pills can be offered if you go to the doctor looking for a quick fix. This potentially can give you temporary relief but usually is not long lasting, as it does not address the root cause of the problem. The best therapy programs will look for why you are having this particular wrist pain and develop a program that will not only get rid of the pain but also find the imbalances and strengthen you, giving you the best chance that it doesn't come back.

A fall or other impact on the wrist might lead to a different type of injury. Our wrist is very complex because it has eight bones which are held together by ligaments. Ligaments are strong and short, holding bone to bone to provide stability. In the wrist, there are a lot of small ligaments that help to ensure our wrist is stable and strong so that our hands have the strength that they need. Any sharp pain at the wrist is worth getting a healthcare professional to take a closer look. If you have fallen or something heavy has fallen onto your wrists, and you have sharp pain with light or moderately heavy things that you are doing, then don't wait. Go to a certified hand therapist to have other problems ruled out and get to the real source of the pain.

Do You Have a Handful of Hand Problems?

Injuries to the hand can be due to fractures from a fall or something over time like a trigger finger. Or both!

What is a trigger finger? Trigger finger is also called tenosynovitis. The best way I can describe it is as having a knot along your tendon. Each finger has two tendons that help pull them into a fist. You also have things called pulleys that hold those tendons down in the palm of your hand where your big knuckles bend. When you develop a knot along that tendon, every time you make a fist, that knot must pass through the pulley system. When you open your fingers, the knot gets stuck and now you must pop it out to straighten the finger. In the process of opening and closing your fingers, that knot – which is swelling – becomes more swollen and irritated. Sometimes it can be the pulley system that gets thick, making it hard for the tendon to pass freely. Both reasons can cause pain. Left untreated, it will become more painful and more difficult to use your hand for any task. Not using the hand will only make it worse by causing stiffness in the fingers, weakness, and more pain. Not all trigger fingers are painful, however. Sometimes it can be loud and hard, and the finger really gets stuck so that the person must manually use the other hand to pull it straight, with no pain at all. Funny how it works, right? The people who we help are the ones who have a painful trigger finger. It can be mild, moderate, or severe. How bad will you let it get before getting help?

I helped one woman who desperately came to our clinic after she had already seen her doctor. Rose asked her primary care doctor what was causing the pain that had been bothering her for months. Her doctor nonchalantly said, "Oh, yes, sounds like a trigger finger. If it bothers you a lot, I can refer you to a hand surgeon for that because you will probably need surgery." Luckily for her, her sister-in-law was a client of ours who was being treated for, among other things, two trigger fingers. Rose didn't want to risk having surgery, so we were able to have her come in for a first session to go over key problems, find solutions, and help her work out the pain and stiffness so that she could

- Have her mind put at ease without jumping into surgery
- Learn what she can do that will fully get rid of the pain and avoid injections and surgery altogether
- Pack for a long-awaited, relaxing, pain-free vacation with her girlfriends – plus enjoy the yoga retreat that she had been looking forward to for months, all without worry

Now that she knew what it was, my client asked, "Why is it happening?" If only it were black and white! It's not always clear why. It can be due to overuse or repetitive use of the hand, or it can be due to an accident like falling on your hand or hitting your hand against something hard. Most slow-to-show type of injuries are not due to something happening yesterday but something that happened months and years ago. That starts a small amount of inflammation which can develop either quickly or slowly over time. It can happen to the thumb (called a trigger thumb) or to any of the fingers, although the two most common are the long and ring fingers. I have seen many patients who unfortunately developed it after surgery to the hand or wrist, who used a prefabricated splint that sits a little too high on the distal palmar crease or who wore the splint longer than they needed. The palm of their hand looks slightly swollen, and the tendons there feel thick. With that kind of wrist, hand, or finger injury, it is common to have swelling and difficulty using your hands and moving your fingers. That sensation of stiffness or pain is usually associated with people consistently opening and closing their fingers only in the limited space where they feel comfortable. This is probably why so many people develop trigger finger as a secondary problem.

Another client came in for our free Discovery Visit complaining of hand pain. Over the phone she didn't recall the name, but in describing her pain and what she was having trouble doing, we knew we could help her and invited her in for our free Discovery Visit. It's an opportunity to talk to her and give her more clarity regarding what kind of help she is seeking. She works as a nail technician, so she is using her hands daily to help others feel good and look good. Nora told us that her hand pain had been bothering her for months (along with elbow and shoulder issues). She got an injection a year or so ago, and its effects lasted a long time. She got another injection after pain started again and would not go away. This time the pain-relieving effect of the cortisone injection lasted only a month. Nora was upset about the effects of the injection not lasting, but her doctor only recommended surgery, the last thing she wanted. Imagine the pain after surgery but also the time and money lost from not being able to work during recovery. In addition, hand therapy is also needed after surgery.

Cortisone injections can help you quickly, but in most cases the pain will return sooner or later. There is nothing wrong with injections if that is what you want. What is not always explained with cortisone injections is that they don't find the root cause of the problem nor do they get rid of the problem altogether. Why do you keep getting trigger fingers or hand pain? If you could get the help you need to get rid of the pain and learn how to keep it from coming back, would you want to do so? If you knew it is 100% possible to avoid trigger finger surgery, would you get the help you needed?

Finger and Thumb Injuries

"Arthritis" of the hand must be the second most common problem I hear of when it comes to the hand. The first is carpal tunnel. Not that everyone has arthritis, but everyone jumps to that conclusion when they have hand or finger pain. There are many forms of arthritis, and it requires a medical doctor to order blood work if you think you are suffering from particular types of arthritis. Depending on the type, there are different solutions involving lifestyle changes and medications. If you do believe you need a doctor's advice for possible arthritis, I recommend you see a rheumatologist who is an expert in arthritis care.

What I am now going to help you understand are "general osteo-arthritis" problems. I'll also provide some solutions if you already know you have some form of arthritis and are seeking help with your pain and mobility to allow you to live more freely with fewer limitations. Osteoarthritis in general describes when there is a change in the joint surface where it is no longer as smooth as it once was. The fluid between your joints, affecting how smoothly everything moves, becomes less and less. This happens as we age, when the feeling of "stiffness" begins to creep in.

The widely held but false belief is that there is nothing that you can do about stiffness because as you get old, you get stiff. However, as you get stiff, you will feel older and older. I know and work with quite a few older clients of ours that are loose, limber, and very active. They do not let the idea of a number slow them down. They continue to work with us in our Wellness Program to keep them mobile and active and avoid pain. I also speak to much younger people who use the same phrases: "I feel old" and "This is happening because I am getting old." I'm not kidding when I say they are in their 20s, 30s, and 40s yet feeling older than those in their 60s, 70s, and 80s!

The common target that gets all the blame is ARTHRITIS! Poor arthritis gets a bad rap. Just because you experience some mild changes doesn't mean you have to live with pain and poor mobility. There are many great things you can do to ensure that your hands work for you for a long time without pain while avoiding injections and surgery.

One of the most common forms of arthritis that I see is arthritis of the thumb, or CMC (carpal metacarpal). It occurs at the base of your thumb at your wrist level. It tends to affect women more than men and often starts after 50 years old. Our thumbs do 50% of the work of our hands, so when thumb pain kicks in, it's quite debilitating, to say the least. With CMC arthritis, it's not only the thumb that can hurt. Because it sits at the wrist level, it affects the wrist as well. Every time you write, use a knife to cut up your food, use chopsticks to eat, open a bottle of water, open the door, or turn the key at your door, you feel the effects of arthritis in the thumb. I don't know of one person that we have helped with CMC arthritis who does not feel utterly frustrated by all the little things that they have trouble doing every day.

Not only does it happen more often in women over 50, it tends to affect both thumbs, not just one. The problem is that women don't know this and tend to ignore the pain and problems that it can bring. There are ways to help reduce the pain and deformity before it gets worse.

We have many small muscles around the thumb that help it move as much as it does. Our thumb can go almost in a full circle – sort of like the shoulder – and because we can move it so much, we sacrifice stability for mobility. The long muscles of the thumb, along with the short, smaller muscles, let us do all that we can inside the hand and allow us not only to have strength but also manipulate small objects.

The base of the thumb, where the CMC joint is located, can get bigger and protrude. It can get red and inflamed. The pain can start as an achiness that doesn't go away. It can be sharp if you try to do something heavy. It might not hurt you all the time, but it can get worse over time, lasting longer and getting stronger. The ball or bony change is there, but that doesn't mean that you can't do anything about it. Of course, you can! It is possible to come for help before you are a step away from surgery or after surgery.

What if you seek help long before surgery? How much better do you think you would feel if you knew you could avoid surgery – or at least delay it?

The appropriate hand therapy clinic can

- Make you a custom-fitted orthosis (splint) that is small and wearable to help support that thumb during painful inflamed times or when doing something involving more weight
- Show you ways to help reduce the pain and achiness
- Teach you techniques and ways in which to protect your thumbs and hands so that they will last longer without surgery

We have a client who came to us for a shoulder problem, and it turned out we also needed to help her with her hands! She explained how her hands were really hurting her and showed me her thumbs. Sandra had been bothered by both her thumbs for the last several years and DID go to a certified hand therapist! That's great, I told her, because I knew she would be getting treatment from another specialized therapist with her best interest at heart. She was very pro-active about protecting her hands. Unfortunately, the custom-made orthoses made for her were not well fitting. We offered to make her some new ones. There are many ways to make an orthosis, using different materials. Sandra agreed, and we made one for her dominant hand. It was made from an ultra-thin but sturdy material with small holes to let her hands breathe. It was low profile, meaning it was small but did the job. She was not only able to feel very comfortable, but it fit like a cozy T-shirt. Her new orthosis reduced her pain while she grabbed her bags or opened doors or grabbed weights for working out, and even when she was practicing yoga. It allowed her to do her everyday activities with less pain. The orthosis is not something that has to be used all the time. It is used when pain flares up, allowing you to keep doing just about everything but protecting the thumbs so the pain can get better. It can be used if you are going to be doing some heavier work where you want to protect it so that the pain doesn't set in. Since her pain has settled, she can work out with weights and do yoga, putting her hands flat without the pain from her thumbs. With bony changes from CMC arthritis, custom-fitted orthoses can be refitted as needed.

Finger Jams and Sprains/Sprains

Ever jam your finger on a door when opening or closing it? Ever reach to catch a ball and jam your finger into it instead of catching it? Ever just move in the wrong way and catch your finger on something? If the sun rises and sets every day, then at some point in your life this has happened. Thankfully, most of the time it is minor. You shake off the pain maybe make a fist and open it to ensure it's not broken, right? I've done it so many times, and I've seen my kids do it repeatedly.

Sometimes in one random moment it can be worse than before. I worked with a gentleman, Jeff, who jammed his finger when he reached to open a door at the same time someone else was opening it. He saw STARS! It was so painful, but he shook it off, opened and closed his hands, and was able to move his fingers. He thought, "That was that. Thankfully it's fine." Only he noticed three or four weeks later that his finger was increasingly painful and getting stiff. He could not make a full fist, and it was bent in a weird angle. He had over time developed what is called a boutonniere deformity. That is when your finger at the middle knuckle is stuck bent down and the little knuckle starts to bend in an upward direction called hyperextension.

I won't lie to you. Once it starts getting stuck like that, it is difficult to fix and is usually painful. At some point you feel frustrated, worried, and at times defeated, thinking it will never get better.

My hope is that I can get to you early, before it gets to that point. Many of our clients whom we have helped with this type of injury tell us that they waited weeks before getting help, researching online, and going to the doctor. All those things are great. We just need you to do it earlier. By the time you notice that this time is NOT like previous times you jammed your fingers, the achiness and pain are lasting a lot longer. Most people just WAIT longer! The hope is that it will be nothing. However, if you're honest, you are worried. Still, it will be weeks before you get to a doctor's appointment. By this time the finger has gotten worse. That's exactly what happened to Jeff and another client of ours, Dan. Dan waited four weeks after he jammed his finger playing basketball.

Did you know that it is possible to access hand therapy before your finger gets stuck? And before you have that appointment with the hand surgeon or primary care doctor, who will refer you to the hand surgeon? I know you might fear the worst and be slow in deciding. Did you know that at our clinic you can come talk to us first before committing time and money? We can give you clarity about the next steps and what you can do to give you peace of mind. One jammed finger can seem so little, yet it can affect other fingers and the rest of your hand. "What if my hand gets stuck like this or get worse?" And the worst-case scenario, "do I need surgery to fix this?" In most cases, no surgery is needed. Hand therapy is the most effective and natural way to have a pain-free hand, prevent deformities and complications, and return you to being active.

Top Tips and Advice

Some of my top tips, if followed, can help you with your hand and wrist pain and how you how to care for our hands without needing a referral from a doctor. At the very least, reading this advice and following these tips can help ease your worries AND your hand pain before spending hours at a doctor's office.

The hand and wrist are intricate and among the most important tools we have at our disposal. We use them so often that we forget how vital it is to keep our hands healthy for their long-term use throughout our lifetime.

Is hand pain interfering with your ability to

- Write or type?
- Open containers or open the door?
- Grab anything heavy?
- Be active in hitting the gym or doing any fitness activity?
- Do everyday things such as playing with your kids or taking care of your family's needs?

Those are just a few examples of how HAND PAIN and WRIST PAIN can interfere with our lives.

Honestly, most people whom I work with tell me that it is not ALWAYS painful but rather achy and annoying and doesn't STOP them from doing anything. However, it does SLOW them down and bothers them more than anything. They also stop doing or doing less of what they want to do. They also WORRY: "What if it gets worse?"

Eventually it does get worse and does stop them. Would you want to know what to do so it doesn't get worse? Do you want to know how you can fix it?

Here are a few tips that can get you started feeling less pain and stopping your hand or wrist from getting worse:

1. **If you are doing anything that causes MORE pain or SHARP pain, please STOP!** At least until you figure it out. I know a lot of people have the "no pain, no gain" mindset, but this is not true when you have hand pain. That applies when you are healthy and back at the gym working out hard, and the "pain" is the pain of effort and exertion. If you are actively looking for help because your hand hurts so much that it worries you, then don't keep aggravating the pain. Figure out what it is, get rid of it, and then do what you love.

2. **A SPECIFIC tip for trigger pain.** If you make a fist or bend your finger to feel or hear the clicking, this ONE thing that I tell you will make the BIGGEST impact on your trigger finger problem. **STOP MAKING IT CLICK.** There is not one person with trigger finger whom I have met or helped who does not constantly move their finger in a way that makes it keep clicking. They do this to double check, "Oh, it is still there," as if it will magically go away on its own. If it is a trigger finger, it usually does not go away on its own. And the more you keep making it click, the WORSE you are making it.

3. **STOP squeezing the ball.** When you ask for help with your hand pain, you might also tell them that your hand feels weak, right? Someone is probably telling you to squeeze the ball. Even the DOCTORS are telling you. It might not be because you are weak, but most likely that your pain makes you FEEL very weak. Squeezing that ball endlessly can cause even more pain later. This is relevant if you have hand or wrist problems or if your fingers are stiff

and they feel stuck. There is a time and place for working on hand strength, but you must get rid of the essential problem before squeezing and squeezing. It might alleviate the problem for the moment, but it usually makes it worse in the long run.

4. **Modify what you are doing.** For example, if you write a lot with the hand that hurts, use a bigger pen or a gel pen so you don't have to press as hard. Using tools that have a bigger handle can also help reduce how much pain you have. These are just a few examples of how you can modify what you are doing. IF you are interested in not having to modify everything that you are doing because of hand pain, I would recommend you find out what is the cause of the hand pain, get to the root cause, and find a solution.

5. **Take frequent breaks.** If your hand hurts, take breaks from what you are doing. For example, if you cook and cut with your painful hand, take breaks so that your hand gets some rest. It's called sustained gripping, meaning that you are holding on for long periods of time. At times that can cause different types of hand pain. It's usually not something that just happened, but something that has built up over time until it suddenly starts to bother you.

6. **Stretch your hand OPEN!** I know that when people have hand pain, they often clench their fist or pump it open and shut. But almost everything we do requires our hand to make a fist, so when you stretch your fingers open and hold them open for a few seconds, that can be very helpful to reducing pain.

7. **Use heat or ice.** Everyone wants to know the BEST thing to do for hand and wrist problems. It all depends on the actual problem. If you have had hand pain for some time now and are not sure what it is – but you want to get started on doing something, anything to help while you decide what to do next – using heat or cold can help your hands feel better in the short term. Which one to use depends on what's going on. I personally like to use heat when my

clients are stiff and use cold when they have muscle pain or swelling. Neither one will hurt you if you use it "incorrectly," but it may not always be the BEST option, depending on what's wrong. If you have a trigger finger or trigger thumb, one of the most effective ways I help our clients reduce the pain and swelling is icing. Not with an ice pack, but with a frozen bottle of water. If you are stiff or have arthritis, heat would be the most soothing, allowing you to stretch to get more motion. It's not a one-size-fits-all, and it's not always the same. The use of heat and ice can change depending on different phases of your recovery.

8. **Give occupational therapy/certified hand therapy a try.** As occupational therapists (OT) and certified hand therapists (CHT), we are uniquely specialized to help clients with all types of hand problems and injuries. So many people don't know how easy it is to access our services. <u>You don't even need a doctor's referral or to talk to your insurance.</u> The first step is talking to us about what worries you, what limits you from being active and pain-free! We also have these amazing workshop events throughout the year (www.handsots.com/workshop) that will give you an opportunity to come learn about what could be wrong and even get your specific questions answered. Avoid letting your hand get worse and the need for pills, injections, and painful surgery by attending one of our events. This allows us get to know you better and to give you clarity regarding your next steps.

I hope these tips help you to get started. If you apply any one of these tips and get a little better, then you will have made my day! I also want you to know that it is ABSOLUTELY POSSIBLE for you to live a quality of life that is more active and pain-free. You don't have to be STUCK. I would love to be able to help you make the right choices for what you need going forward so that aches don't turn into debilitating pain and the need for surgery. You get to choose how you move forward.

Chapter 6

Stuck on Elbows

Who gets elbow pain, why, and why they are stuck for so long?
Who gets elbow pain?

J UST ABOUT EVERYONE has elbow pain at some point in their life. It's a common problem! It's just not always talked about, at least not in a way that tells you that you can get help. I see both men and women with elbow pain. On the web you'll find plenty of talk about sports injuries, but regular people like you and me can experience elbow pain while doing everyday things such as working, grocery shopping, or taking care of your home and family. No one thing causes elbow pain.

Here are some very common elbow problems that we see at Hands-On Therapy Services:

- Tendinitis (both inside and outside the elbow, also known as golfer's elbow and tennis elbow respectively)
- Nerve problems at the elbow area
- Arthritis of the elbow
- Fractures and other surgeries at the elbow area

I'm sure if you have an elbow problem, you have already Googled "tennis elbow." You'll be told to go to a doctor if you are experiencing excruciating pain. In the worst-case scenario, such as after a fall, then yes, you must go to the emergency room or your doctor. In most other cases, elbow problems such as tendinitis tend to creep up on you. It aches here and there for a few days, and then it's gone. "Great," you think. "I don't need to waste time and money going to the doctor. Let's be honest, what are they going to tell me anyway?" All my friends and clients with elbow problems tell me that's what they were thinking.

What is tendinitis?

Lateral epicondylitis (also known as tennis elbow) and medial epicondylitis (golfer's elbow) are the degeneration (little tears) of specific areas of the tendons at the elbow. Lateral is the outside of the elbow and medial is the inside of the elbow. The most common is the lateral or tennis elbow tendinitis. It's a small, strong muscle of the forearm that steadies your wrist when using your hand. Sometimes, it's from overuse or doing the same thing over and over. It's not just ONE muscle – even though one muscle does have a bad rap. It's usually a group of muscles that are painful, tight, and problematic.

If you have elbow pain on the INSIDE of your elbow, it's called medial epicondylitis. It's just the name of the location. You may have inflammation at the tendon area or tight muscles. It's also known as golfer's elbow, even though you may never have swung a golf club!

What stops people from getting help?

If your elbow was bothering you, perhaps you talked to a friend or family member. What did they tell you? They will most likely tell you one of these things THEY did or didn't do to make their elbow pain go away:

- Do nothing because the pain will go away if you rest your arm
- Buy a forearm brace/wrap and wear it
- Take anti-inflammatory pills like Advil or Aleve
- Go to the doctor for an injection

To do nothing

The elbow pain MIGHT go away for good. For most people, it may get a little better. For some, because the pain is not STOPPING them, it's hard to make time to take care of the elbow. This type of tendinitis creeps up on you. At first, there's an ache, and then it goes away, but it comes back. At some point the pain is very bad, so most people start to take it more seriously and consider going to the doctor for advice or researching what they can do on their own.

Most of our clients wait until the pain is unbearable. They can't take it anymore. It's either stopping them from doing something that they want to do or it's really slowing them down. Tennis elbow has become golfer's elbow and vice versa. Everything hurts. They didn't know that occupational therapy is an option to help them with the pain, heal the area, and teach them how to take care of their elbow and arm.

What about wearing the forearm wrap or brace?

Almost ALL our clients ask about the forearm brace. These bracing companies want to tell you what you want to hear – that this ONE brace can fix all your pain. Doctor's offices sell them like candy, and it's found at all pharmacies. I get it. It's easy, fast, and cheap. It might reduce the pain somewhat so that you think the problem is fixed. One of our clients told me he had been wearing a brace for 15 YEARS! It provides temporary relief but only masks the problem. The pain would come back when he started any activity. Then he would put on his brace, and it would feel less painful. He was wearing it when he came to our clinic. Ask yourself this: do you want to merely mask the elbow problem, or do you want to heal it so it won't keep coming back?

Taking anti-inflammatory pills

Anti-inflammatory pills can decrease pain and, if taken correctly, can reduce the swelling in your body. The pills help the whole body, not just your arm. It can take awhile to help with elbow pain. This can be difficult for someone who is already taking pills and doesn't want to take MORE pills, who wants to reduce pain naturally, or who has pill-caused stomach problems. Usually the pills take the edge off the pain. But the long-term use of pills is bad for you. All meds have side effects. I know firsthand from my husband, who used to take Advil all the time for his migraines, that it can lead to heart issues. There's always a time and place for pain medications, but why take pills when you know there are other options to take care of your elbow pain?

If you are suffering from elbow pain, yes, you can go to the doctor

Doctors will tell you to rest your arm, write a prescription for stronger anti-inflammatory pills or muscle relaxers. Few recommend therapy, whether it be physical therapy or occupational therapy. Fewer recommend a Certified Hand Therapist who specializes in arm and hand problems. Even when doctors do recommend therapy, many of our clients tell us they wait so long because it was "not that bad" or they "didn't know where to go."

Most people suffering from elbow pain go to the doctor already having done some research. They'll say, "I know I have tennis elbow, right?" They will wait for the doctor to say, "YES, that's it, here are some pills to take." If it's bad, the doctor will give you an injection of cortisone to rid you of the pain. That's fastest, easiest option. For some people, it works, and hopefully the effects will last for years. For most, injections don't provide lasting relief from pain, so another injection will be recommended. If you're not free from pain for at least six months, injections don't work for you. A general rule of thumb is no more than two or three injections in the same part of the body.

PRP injections, a relatively new procedure, can also be tried. It injects your own blood into the damaged area of your elbow. It's almost like having a surgery in how they prep you. You may need two or three procedures to get the results you seek.

Surgery to the elbow for tennis elbow is not a common procedure. It's the LAST option if you have already tried specialized therapy services and injections but nothing has worked. During surgery the damaged tissues are scraped. Recovery, including therapy, can take upwards of six months.

What's STOPPING you?

What STOPS people from getting help isn't a lack of options. It's that there are **too many options** and voices trying to help. Going to the doctor? Past clients have told me they go, get the confirmation that it is tendinitis, are offered pills, injection, and possibly referred to therapy services. But which therapy clinic? What would actually help?

Most people with elbow pain or elbow problems can live without pain and limitations by getting conservative treatments. The problem is that most people get STUCK thinking that elbow pain will get better on its own. Or they think they can get rid of it by themselves. Or they try to rest it by not using their arm as much.

If you want to avoid injections and surgery and eliminate pain naturally, my best recommendation is not to wait. It's possible to rid yourself of that elbow achiness and avoid wearing a forearm brace or taking pills. If you've never had any kind of therapy before, you may not know what to expect.

If you have tried therapy before and didn't get the results you were hoping for, I can understand why you hesitate to try again. Don't be stuck in a general therapy clinic, doing the same exercises over and over without getting rid of the aches and pain.

Either way, I would highly recommend that you speak to us first. Let's get clear about what you are looking for and what may be possible to help you get rid of your pain. If not us, then look for a therapy clinic in your area where you can speak with the specialist first to figure out what type of program they have that can benefit you.

My most recent client came to us after suffering elbow pain for several months. She didn't have tremendous pain that stopped her from doing her normal activities, but she was worried that it might come to that eventually. She is a musician who earns her income using her arms. With the elbow pain she was experiencing, it made it difficult to work as much as she wanted. She had engagements and commitments. What if one day her arms were very painful? Not only would she lose out on work right now, but if people saw her as not being reliable, it would be more difficult to get future work. By the time she came to our free Discovery Visit, she was really disheartened about the whole therapy process. Would it help her? She was not interested in getting injections from a doctor. She wanted to get rid of the pain and learn how to have more control over it in the future if it were to occur again. As a musician, she will need her arms to be able play for as long as possible.

She knew after a few short months that rest was not making the elbow pain better, so she sought out professional help. She went to a doctor who recommended therapy at their own facility. It was a well known place. They treated her nicely enough, and she could use her insurance. She did all the right things and was still frustrated and feeling defeated. When she called us, we were her last hope. I could hear her frustration, and I knew she was skeptical about doing business with us. After our conversation, she sounded like someone that we could help so I invited her to our free Discovery Visit. It was a great way for us to meet and a safe, RISK-FREE way for her to get to know us and learn if we TRULY could solve her problem.

I can't tell you enough how much I loved working with her! We were able to make sure that we were a good fit and could meet her needs before taking her on as a client. She was able to know that we were invested in her as much as she was in herself. With a very specific plan developed just for her, we were able to increase her play time as a musician from 30 minutes to two hours plus without pain or fatigue. She was able to get back to yoga and barre classes and go to the gym to stay healthy and fit. She was even able to fix herself one day when she felt some discomfort during an extended session. She sent an email, and I was able to remind her of one part of her program that she had forgotten. BAM! She fixed herself before she came in for her last session. We gave her exactly what she wanted in a time frame that worked for her. Busy season comes and goes in the music world, and now she is ready. Not only did we get rid of her discomfort, but we set her up to help herself in the future. The BEST part was that she was happy and worry-free after the help we gave her. Nothing is better for me than helping someone lift their spirits.

What you can do to get started

Elbow pain is one of those things that begins, goes away when you rest, and comes back. It's not from any ONE thing that you did but rather an accumulation of wear over time. We use our arms for everything, and sometimes they hurt.

Most people tell me that elbow pain is more a "discomfort" than a true "pain." It can become more painful over time, but it tends to be achy and annoying. It slows you down more than stopping you. Most people just live with it and power through. It's not the same as if you fell and broke the bones of your elbow and had to have surgery (but we will talk about that later).

Here are a few things that you can do if you think you have tennis elbow or golfer's elbow – any type of elbow – "itis." These are my favorite tips to give to my clients. They involve modifying your body mechanics while doing things to PREVENT it from getting worse.

1. **If you are doing anything that causes MORE pain or SHARP pain, please STOP!** It seems like such a simple thing you are doing, but all of the sudden you get a sharp pain that radiates down your hand and makes you want to drop what you're holding. The sharpness goes away, but you know it won't be for long. I know a lot of people have the "no pain, no gain" mindset, but this is not true when you have elbow or arm pain. Reserve that for when you're healthy and back at the gym doing a hard workout. Take caution when that pain becomes sharp. Don't keep aggravating the pain.

2. **Stop squeezing the ball.** I know when you ask for help with your elbow pain, you might also tell them that your hand feels weak, right? And someone is telling you to squeeze the ball. Even the DOCTORS are telling you. It might not be because you are weak but most likely that your pain makes you feel very weak. Squeezing that ball endlessly can likely cause more pain because the muscles that move your wrist and hand start at the elbow. Squeezing the ball can continue to irritate the tendons even though you don't feel it right away.

3. **Modify what you are doing.** Heavy gripping to carry bags or other objects can also aggravate that pain. I think carrying grocery bags are the WORST when there is elbow pain! We have a sustained grip on bags that can get very heavy because we want to carry everything on the first trip into the house (you know what I'm talking about!). We do it with our palms down, and when we put the groceries on the counter, we are reaching with the arm away from our body. This can strain muscles that are already tight and irritate tendons that are already inflamed. If you have elbow

pain while working out, try not to hold heavy weights for a long time with a tight grip. I see white knuckles from people holding so tightly. Try other workouts like using a machine that doesn't require sustained gripping. Keep your wrist straight and stable while working out with other parts of your body.

4. **Modify body mechanics.** When carrying anything heavy, hold it close to your body instead of with your arms stretched out in front of you. When carrying something heavy, hold it with your palms up, not down. If your elbow hurts after typing a lot, give more support to your arms so that your shoulders and wrists are not overworking. These simple tips can help you while you are in pain and keep you from continuing to irritate your elbow.

5. **Limit any sustained gripping or squeezing.** That means holding on to something for a long time. For instance, when cleaning, squeezing out a sponge, or cutting a lot of meat and veggies. Not saying you can't do it. Just give yourself breaks to avoid a flare-up. If you are like me – and most every person – we want to start it and just get done already!

6. **Stretch it often!** I know when people have arm pain, one of the things they do is clench their fist or pump it open and shut. Honestly, everything we do requires our arms so make sure to stretch the WHOLE arm, from the hands all the way to the shoulders. Hold it for 10-15 seconds. That can be very helpful in reducing your pain. Did you know that when your elbow hurts, it could be something from your shoulder or from your wrist? A specific strengthening program will help not only to reduce the pain, but ensure your best chances of not having elbow pain come back. Stretching is a great place to start but don't get stuck there.

7. **Use ice.** If you have had pain for some time now and you're not sure what it is, but you want to get started doing something, anything, to help while you decide what you can do next, using ice can help your elbow feel better in the short term. Ice both the outside and inside parts of your elbow

and forearm. The inside of your elbow is more sensitive, but you can do it. It may be uncomfortable at first, but as it gets numb, you won't feel a thing. And ice has the benefit of lasting for up to two hours after you take it off. I'm asked, "Why not heat?" My answer is to use heat if you are feeling stiff and just because it feels good. But its effects are not as long-lasting or effective as ice when it comes to tendinitis.

8. **Massage around the area of pain**. Massage the bone bump on both the inside and outside of your elbow. Make sure to massage ABOVE and BELOW. Get to those tight and sometimes painful muscles! They just need a little tender loving care.

9. **Take pills?** Usually doctors will recommend taking some type of anti-inflammatory medication to help with the pain. If you are not taking it consistently, it is just a painkiller and not helping to reduce the deep swelling that is inside your arm. I always caution my clients to beware if they have stomach issues.

Follow these tips to ease some of your elbow discomfort or pain. I hope these tips help you get started feeling better and decide how to have a more active and pain-free way of living. You may ask, why do I need to slow down or take frequent breaks for my elbow or why can't I do certain things because I know that it will hurt me? The answer is there. There's professional help for people suffering with elbow problems.

Why is it happening to me?

How much you are using your arms and HOW you are using them play a role, too. Sometimes it just takes one tweak that's weird to create an imbalance. More and more I am finding that people with prolonged elbow issues have shoulder or hand problems. Who knows which came first. I know the most important thing is getting to the root cause of the problem in order to get rid of the pain, fix the imbalance, and provide strengthening. That will give you the best possible chance of elbow pain not returning any time soon.

Have you tried those tips above, yet need a little more? We want to help you get clarity on what you can do next to rid yourself of elbow pain. I have videos that may help you. At the very least, reading this elbow chapter can give you some insight into what is possible, starting with the tips that can help ease your elbow pain before spending hours at a doctor's office. I even have some videos that you may find helpful on our Hands-On Therapy Services YouTube channel. Arms are intricate and are among the most important tools that we have at our disposal. It's vital to keep our arms healthy for long-term use.

Can therapy REALLY help, though?

The right therapy can help! Of course, just like anything else, not all therapists and therapy centers are cut from the same cloth. No matter how long you have been suffering with tendinitis, it is possible to get rid of the pain and problems in your elbow. If you have listened to friends and family say, "Oh, I have suffered for years, and it's not possible to get rid of it," then let me be the first person to tell you they're WRONG! If you've gone to other therapy centers but didn't get better, don't let that experience taint the possibility of recovery. How much better you want to be and how committed you are to the plan and to finding the root cause of the problem determine how much better you will get.

I have battled my own personal fight with tennis elbow. I developed it years ago when I switched from one job setting to another. I had been an acute care occupational therapist at a hospital. I provided therapy for sick patients in the hospital or for those who had surgery but were not medically ready to be discharged. I moved from that position to one in the outpatient therapy department. The people there needed therapy but could come and go.

Switching jobs meant changing what I did daily. In an acute care hospital setting, I walked a lot because it was a large, 500-bed hospital, and I did a lot of heavy lifting. Patients were sick or recovering from surgery and could not get in and out of bed by themselves. They needed to be re-taught how to do the basics of taking care of themselves. Therefore, the work was much heavier. In the outpatient setting, it was easier on my back because clients could come in and leave on their own. Even if they were in a wheelchair, I didn't have to do any heavy lifting. I mostly helped people with arm and hand injuries. I would use both my hands to stretch tight and stiff fingers, wrist, elbows, and shoulders. There was a lot more paperwork, too. Plus, it was the three-sheet, carbon-copy-type of paper documentation, so I really had to press down on the page.

I quickly started tiredness in my hands and forearms. They would be tight while I was cleaning the house or making dinner. That's when it happened! I was squeezing out a sponge and – BAM! The sharp, electric pain started at my elbow and shot down my arm. I had to drop the sponge! It was crazy how painful it was for a split second. Afterwards I had a dull ache that went away after resting it. But when was I going to rest it? In my sleep? Back to work I went. It was not hurting all the time, only on random occasions. I figured it would go away on its own. I KNEW it was tennis elbow, but I wasn't doing what I needed to get rid of it for good.

I needed to find the root cause of the problem. Does it mean I will never get tennis elbow again? If I clean my car once, does it mean it will be clean forever? I wish! But no. I can't STOP using my arms to help others have pain-free arms. Finding out the root cause of my pain allowed me to know what I needed to do to get rid of my elbow pain and strengthen my elbow specifically so it doesn't become painful again. I don't want to be limited, and I don't want you to be limited. We can help you get rid of your elbow pain, too. It just takes commitment to wanting to be pain-free.

How do I know it's a nerve problem at the elbow?

Are you having any numbness and tingling in your hand? Not just to any fingers but to your small finger and ring finger? It comes and goes, but it's uncomfortable. That's how it starts. Then it can become painful. Not the pain that's sharp. It's more of an achy, sensitive kind of pain. The numbness is the worst feeling. You can lose sensation in your fingers, making you feel weak and clumsy. Leave it untreated and it can become painful at the elbow, with numbness that is constantly there.

Ever notice when it happens? Do you have it at certain times? Does it happen when you wake up in the morning or when you are lying down in a certain position OR when you are holding the phone to your ear? If so, you may be experiencing some ulnar nerve problems (aka Cubital Tunnel). It is most common at the elbow, where the "funny bone" is. When you accidentally hit the inside area of your elbow, there's a sharp fiery pain and tingling that radiate down your arm to your fingers. That's the ulnar nerve.

When you are having tingling on the pinky side of your hand, your ulnar nerve may be irritated either at your neck/shoulder area, elbow area, or wrist area. Everyone always thinks it's "carpal tunnel," because there has been a lot of recent talk about carpal tunnel. However, it's VERY important to know which nerve is irritated so that we can get you the best possible treatment.

It's common in pregnant women as the body changes, but usually goes away after having the baby. It can happen to anyone, but in my years of helping people with elbow pain, I do notice it in woman more than in men. The literature says that it may happen in women more than men because our bodies may have smaller canals and structures that increase the chances of these types of issues. The nerve may be irritated or compressed in certain positions and with certain activities.

Nerves don't move like muscles move but they still need to move a little bit. They need to glide around and respond well to tension. When there's an injury or not enough of the right kind of movement, scarring can develop around very specific areas where the nerve passes. In the case of cubital tunnel, it most commonly gets trapped at the elbow level. It can also be at the neck and wrist level and still make your fingers numb and tingle, so it's so important to get to the root cause of what is going wrong so that you can fix it in the best way.

Some helpful tips for your Cubital Tunnel Syndrome

1. **That nerve is most compressed when your elbow is bent!** The ulnar nerve is already stuck around that elbow area and not moving well. When you keep your elbow bent, it compresses the nerve even more. For example, if you are having numbness on your pinky side of your hand when holding the phone up to your ear for a few minutes, you are overstretching and pressing on that nerve. Try switching hands often or using an earpiece.

2. **That nerve is compressed if you are putting direct pressure on it!** The ulnar nerve is the most sensitive nerve that you have. Hence, the funny bone hurts and shoots electric feelings down your hand when you hit that corner of your elbow. If you have numbness when falling asleep or when you wake up, it could be how you are lying down. If you are sleeping on your back and the elbows are pressing into the mattress, that could be pressing on that nerve. The easiest thing you can do is place a pillow under your arm so that it lifts the elbow off the bed a little. Or it could be that you are curled up into a ball so that your elbow is completely bent. Well, the elbow can't be fully bent like that for too long. Otherwise, it will press on that nerve. One thing you can do is wrap the elbow with a thick towel to keep it

from bending all the way in. If you are a left-handed writer, this may become an issue for you because your positioning may put pressure on the ulnar nerve when writing.

These are just two MAIN problems with the nerve at the elbow area, with a few tips on what you can quickly do on your own to ease that numbness and irritation. In my experience, most people wait and wait because it's not excruciating pain or not numb all the time. By the time they go to the doctor, though, the pain can be bad. Most doctors do some of the following:

- Usually recommend a splint or a brace that is used at night. Most people find using the splint at night to sleep is too uncomfortable. A soft brace may help, but it doesn't always fit well or restrict the motion that you need to restrict. Sometimes it works, and sometimes it doesn't
- Often recommend taking pills
- Sometimes recommend a nerve conduction test
- Frequently tell you to wait until the pain is so bad that you will qualify for surgery.

If you are looking to avoid surgery, let's look at what could be happening above and below the elbow, so we can get to the root cause. When I talk to people with this elbow problem, where numbness goes down to the hand, I always seem to find that it's more than one thing. It could be that the muscles around the area are tight. Sometimes I find that the shoulder and neck are the troublemakers and that the muscles around them are tight as well. They just need hands-on work to get them loose.

If you are having numbness and tingling on your pinky side of your hands – AND you are invested in your health and looking for more natural ways of healing – then just know that there are alternatives for getting better. It is possible to get rid of it completely. Don't wait for it to get worse before acting. If you want great quality sleep and want to use your hands and arms without any pain or numbness, and if you want to avoid surgery, then request to speak to one of our specialists to help you get some clarity.

Natural, conservative treatment is the BEST way of getting rid of cubital tunnel syndrome. However, there is ONE instance where I tell a potential client that, no, I can't take you on as a client and I need you to consult with a surgeon (though it still all depends). When you have cubital tunnel syndrome but have waited so long before seeking help that you have signs of atrophy in your hands, that is a clear sign that you may need surgery.

Occasionally I work with someone who has atrophy but can't have surgery. They know the limitations of the results that we can achieve. Having the nerve compressed so much for so long, the nerves can no longer send signals for the muscles to work. The muscles start to waste away, resulting in atrophy. Once you are at that point, even with surgery it's difficult to say that you will recover completely. Surgery is necessary to make sure that you don't get worse, and it will help with the sensation of numbness and pain or achiness.

I urge you not to wait. Nerves are complicated. Once there is nerve death from being compressed too long, you can't go back in time to reverse the damages completely. Even if you don't come to Hands-On Therapy Services, please consider going somewhere to get the help that you need so that it doesn't get worse. I hear the "I wish I didn't wait so long" from so many of my clients. I understand that sometimes you are just not ready. But in terms of nerve problems, such as cubital tunnel, at least get some questions answered so that you can be clear on what to do next.

Common fractures and other surgeries to the elbow

Picture this: you are doing great. Loving life. Getting more active and hitting your fitness goals. Work is good. Maybe even great, as you were just promoted or doing your own thing and hustling. Then shit hits the fan. You were biking, and in a freak moment you fell onto your outstretched hands. You were on a ladder taking care of some trees. You were just walking or running. Life happens. You break your elbow. Then what comes next?

Your elbow has three bones: distal humerus, radial head, and ulna. Which one did you break, how many of them did you break, and how bad was it? Did you need surgery or not? When this happens, the first thing you do is go to the Emergency Room. Or Urgent Care. They can determine if you broke bones and how badly. If it was determined that something is broken but not life threatening, then you get placed with one of those bulky casts that is wrapped up tight to stabilize your elbow. You are then placed in a sling and sent home with instructions to follow up with an orthopedic surgeon. If your elbow is broken so badly that you need surgery right away (this may depend on where you go), then the orthopedic surgeon on call will most likely be the one to operate.

In your desperation, you don't care who's doing your surgery as long as someone can fix your arm. I hope you do get to pick who does your surgery, though. People who come to me after surgery often ask, "Did I have a good surgeon?" Listen, there are very few bad surgeons, plenty of good ones, and a few GREAT ones. I've always said, almost everything in life falls on a bell curve. Surgeons are no different. Who do you want to do your surgery if you can have a choice?

It doesn't matter if your surgeon has a favorite therapy center or maybe his or her own that they funnel their patients into. You DO get to pick WHO helps you after your surgery. Even with surgeons who recommend Hands-On Therapy Services after a patient's surgery, we always talk to them to make sure we're a good fit with respect to their goals. We like to work with people who are as committed as we are in getting the BEST possible results from their surgery.

What happens next?

Now that your elbow is stabilized, either with a cast or surgery, what happens next? The most important thing I want you to know about elbows after a fracture or surgery is that elbows like to MOVE. They get stuck very easily and, once stuck, it's very hard to reach for everything that we take for granted: touching your face or mouth, grabbing a door, reaching for a glass, turning a key, or washing your face. The elbow helps to bring your hands to and from your body.

There is a general protocol concerning when you are suppose to start therapy and how you should progress. It's very important to know what happened to you and whether your injury is "stable." That just means that everything's in its place. It is difficult to remember to ask your doctors all these questions. Lots of people forget what they wanted to ask. There's so much to remember that you can't recall all the answers. Being in excruciating pain doesn't help! Talk to your therapist who specializes in elbow injuries.

For instance, if you had a radial head fracture in your elbow that was very small, most doctors will not cast you. They will place you in a sling and tell you to start moving. If it's worse (ie. not stable), they may place you in a cast, but it should not be on for more than two or three weeks. Elbows get extremely stiff and can become very hard to move in both directions.

My husband fell and broke his radial head years ago. He was playing tennis with my brother when a huge lightning storm quickly rolled up right over them. Lightning struck very close by, which set my husband running. He tried to jump over the net in his hurry to leave. He's tall but not very athletic. He caught the tip of his shoe on the top of the net and tumbled to the ground with arms stretched out. BOOM! Pain shot up his arm when he fell. He was able to pick himself up, and they headed out of the park. He thought it was only his ego that was bruised, but by the time he got home, he was in a lot of pain and could not move his arm. We iced it and decided to go the Emergency Room for X-rays. Sure enough, there was a very small fracture, but at least it was not displaced, as the bones were still together. The following day, we were able to see an orthopedic surgeon, who removed the temporary cast they placed on him in the ER and left him with a sling. Because the fracture was so small, the elbow was stable. The most important thing to do was start moving. It hurt like hell.

I was just starting out as a therapist then, and we had no kids. I thought, "Sure, I'll be your therapist." Let me tell you that doing therapy on your spouse, especially in the beginning stages of an injury, is NOT the best decision. I now KNOW from my experience and the experience of others whom I have seen try. After one month (for the sake of our marriage), we decided that he needed to be seen by a Certified Hand Therapist. It's hard to have to hurt the person that you love. It's also hard to make the time that is needed CONSISTENTLY to get the results that I know he wanted. It is great to be the cheerleader, to be the support person but difficult to be the full-time therapist and spouse or family member.

If you need surgery to fix broken bones, once that fracture is stable from the surgery you should start therapy right away. I used to work with a surgeon at Mount Sinai, where five days post-operation I would remove the post-op dressing, make sure the incision was healing well, and start moving the elbow. Since then, I've worked with other surgeons who want their patients to wait a bit longer before starting to move. Either way, ask your surgeon what their protocol is OR ask US what the protocol should be after your fracture or surgery. We can help you determine what that protocol is based on your surgery. And because we work with so many surgeons in the Miami/Fort Lauderdale area, we know the protocols of the various doctors. If we don't, it's easy for us to get on the phone with their office to obtain the information we need to help you understand what happened to you and help you know the next steps.

Depending on the elbow surgery, some are allowed to start right away. By right away, I mean within three to five days after a fracture. Once you follow up with the surgeon to remove the post-op dressing, you should start therapy on your elbow. It's BEST if you start researching where you want to go for your elbow therapy even if you don't have the dressing off yet, because it may take you a few days to get an appointment. At our clinic, we try our hardest to give priority to the first session after surgery. We KNOW what a major difference in results our clients experience when they start therapy right away versus waiting. We also talk with our clients first to determine, based on their surgery, when is the best time to get started. We know and understand that some people are scared. They have no pain, and they don't want to do anything to damage their surgery. Some people don't know and think they must wait until the stitches are out, but they don't have to wait. It is in your best interest to get started earlier rather than later. And if not to get started, at least to call and talk to our specialist to know WHEN is the best time to get started.

After knowing when to get started, our next most common question we are asked is, "Will I recover fully?" That is one of the hardest questions to answer. There are too many factors involved. What was broken or damaged? Who did the surgery and when? When did you start therapy? Where are you going for your therapy? How committed are you to getting the results that you want?

The ONLY thing that is important and that YOU have control over and are able to decide is, "Where are you deciding to go for your therapy?" Are you going to a clinic where the therapist puts you and your goals first? Are you going to a clinic where you are getting the time and attention that you need to work toward that full recovery? Are you going to a clinic where you are receiving support while you are there as well as when you are not?

Injuries like falls and surgeries are difficult and time sensitive. Who you choose to work with is important. In the case of my husband, he (we) decided it was best for him to get outside help. But if I knew then what I know now, I truly believe that he would have a straight elbow. He can do everything, no issues, but he never got FULL motion straightening his elbow. I attribute that to not paying enough attention to him and his paid therapy. I remember when he came home and told me his therapist decided that after four weeks he was done and could do everything on his own. I firmly believe that most of us need more help to stay accountable and stay on task. He sits and works on a computer for God's sake! That keeps your elbows bent all day! Therefore, finding out what he does all day, what he is wanting and expecting from therapy, and what he can actually do himself are very important aspects of helping him determine the best plan of action.

For people who have radial head fractures that do not require surgery, it is very possible to get 100 percent of their function and motion without pain. It does require a commitment on your part and our part to help you stay accountable and keep making the progress you desire.

A client of mine several years ago fell while running and broke both of his elbows. One side was fractured at the radial head and only needed to be casted. The other radial head required surgery. He was in the cast for about three weeks, but the side that had surgery was out of the post-op dressing and was in a custom-fitted orthosis for protection. He was able to start moving the side with the surgery right away. Even though there was pain, we were able to have him manage it while reaching his goals. Considering that both his arms were broken he couldn't use his other hand to help. When he first came to us, he literally couldn't do anything. He couldn't feed himself, go to the bathroom or bathe himself. Not even scratch an itch on his nose. These are everyday activities that we take for granted. In a split second it was gone, at least temporarily. By the time he was done with therapy, he was able to move fully and do it all himself. He even put some weight through his arms to push himself off the floor, play with his little kids, and strengthen his arms at the gym. We were able to take him as far as he needed to go because we found what was most important for the best possible results not just immediately but in the future as well. He wanted to be able to play with his kids and not feel restricted. And he didn't want to be careful because his arms didn't move well or because of pain. Asking him all the right questions, we were able to develop an action plan to meet his needs.

Elbow injuries that involve a fracture or surgery can be difficult. You should know that it's POSSIBLE to get the best results when you understand what is going on and what is at stake: your full recovery with the least complications your ability to feel great now and in the future when you are committed to your recovery. If you had an elbow injury – whether recently or months ago – and you are wondering if you can get help to get the best recovery from your injury, request to speak to our specialist and get clarity on what you can do next.

Chapter 7

Shouldering Through the Pain

Common shoulder problems –
tendinitis, bursitis, rotator cuff tears,
impingement, frozen shoulder

WAS TALKING WITH a client who came to our clinic for shoulder problems. His wife is a friend and fellow occupational therapist. She had been telling me for months that her husband was having shoulder issues, but she couldn't convince him to schedule an appointment for just one session or even a Discovery Visit to meet and discuss what help he could use. Only after his shoulder problem interrupted his workout routine did he decide to come for advice. His online research suggested he might have a rotator cuff tear, but he wasn't sure. He said he thought it was because he was getting old. He was just over 40.

Having shoulder problems and
not sure what to do about it?

Shoulder issues making you feel old? You are not alone. Just about everyone who has shoulder problems tells me this. No matter the age, pain and limitations remind us of how we used to feel and what we once were able to do. However, we can change that.

At some point most people face these common shoulder problems: tendinitis, bursitis, impingement, rotator cuff tears, and frozen shoulder, to name a few. Shoulder problems tend to become more prevalent after the age of 40 due to wear and tear.

Tendinitis or bursitis of the shoulder is a very common diagnosis that describes inflammation of the tendon or the bursa, which is a fat pad. There can also be degeneration, which just means there is fraying or small tears in that area. Depending on the severity, it can be painful all the time or only with certain movements. Usually it's painful with motion and can limit you from doing the simplest movements, such as reaching overhead or behind you.

Shoulder impingement is when the two bones of the shoulder keep hitting together and pinching the tendons between. It's not just an ache but a sharp pain when the bones hit together, radiating down the arm. Impingement can cause tendinitis and vice versa. Impingements that are not taken care of can, over time, cause rotator cuff tears.

Rotator cuff tears vary depending on what's going on and how the injury occurred. We have four muscles that make up the rotator cuff. Their purpose is to keep the ball in the socket of the shoulder so that you can maintain shoulder stability. You can tear part of the rotator cuff if you are manipulating something heavy. It can also happen if you grab something hard to prevent falling. There are tons of traumatic ways that rotator tendons can tear. However, tendons are strong, and tears usually occur in a way involving something strong or heavy. Rotator cuff tendons can also tear a little bit over time.

Think about it. To use our hands, our shoulders must place our arms in space and move them around so that we can do everything from getting dressed to cutting up and eating our food. There's not much you can do without your shoulders. Our shoulders themselves are considered "unstable." That means that for us to be able to move our arms around as much as we do, the ball is bigger than the socket, so it relies on the muscles and tendons to hold it together. That's different from our hips. Because our hips don't have as much range of motion, the socket is bigger than the ball, giving the hips more stability.

Because of how much mobility our shoulders have, we sacrifice stability. Therefore, at some point in your life, your shoulders will likely give you some trouble. It's our job to take care of our shoulders so that we can use them without pain and avoid rotator cuff tears.

Research shows that, after the age of 40, we tend to have some wear and tear of the rotator cuff tendons. However, that doesn't always mean that there are tears and pain that would require surgery. As a matter of fact, some people have small tears and don't even know it, don't have pain, and are not limited in what they want to do. Small tears are usually treated conservatively, without surgery. If the tendon is fully torn, then surgery is recommended. Of course, that is also age dependent and based on activity level.

Frozen shoulder is not as simple as the shoulder getting stuck. There are two ways to develop frozen shoulder. A true "adhesive capsulitis" is when you literally wake up from one day to the next with extreme pain. That pain is constant and stops you from moving, which causes the joint to get stuck. There are several phases to it, and therapy can help.

The other way is the most common way people think about frozen shoulder. If you hurt your shoulder and then unconsciously or consciously decide not to use your shoulder fully because of pain, then over a short period of time the shoulder joint itself gets stiff and stuck. You end up with a frozen shoulder. It can be painful all the time or it can be painful when you try to move it. Either way, there is pain when lifting over your head or trying to sleep. The longer your shoulder cannot move fully, the more limited you will feel. Frozen shoulder can also develop after a surgery due to pain, if you don't move your shoulder as much as it needs to move.

Why do people have shoulder problems and what stops them from getting help?

Shoulder problems can develop at ANY age! I've worked with plenty of people who develop shoulder problems in their 20s, 30s, and beyond. I'm not talking about people who fall and break their arms or are in accidents that require surgery. I'm referring to people who are trying to live their best life and, because of their work or particular body type, tend to have shoulder problems.

However, most people who talk to us about their shoulder problems are over 40. Research shows that normal wear and tear starts to manifest itself after age 40. It doesn't mean that once you are 40 it's all downhill from there! But the longer you wait the more wear and tear will build up. How bad do you want to let your shoulder problems become?

Why wait for the help you need? I've asked that of plenty of people we have helped in addition to friends and family. I can tell you with certainty that there are two groups of people:

The first and larger group of people start to have shoulder pain here and there, but for the most part it's not all the time and doesn't stop them from doing anything. They are not concerned even if the pain has been there for months or even years. They do think about it. It does slow them down or makes them feel stiff. Perhaps they must be more careful with certain motions. Maybe they stop doing a specific task. But the pain is manageable with pills. They may worry that it can get worse, but since it hasn't, they choose to wait (P.S. I have tons of these stories).

The other, smaller group tends to get help faster when they have shoulder problems that don't resolve themselves in a few weeks. They don't want to wait until the pain gets worse or until it stops them from doing what they want to do.

Oh, there's a third group. They no longer can wait. Once the pain is constant or once they can't lift their arms to do simple tasks such as dressing or brushing their hair, there is no waiting. They want help and the only thing stopping them is where to go. We are grateful when they trust in us to help them.

Which group are you in? Not sure if therapy can help you? Not sure where to go? Keep reading to get some tips that I share with our clients.

The downside of waiting, the upside of knowing when to get help

Is there a downside to waiting? Yes. We spoke to a gentleman who was clearly frustrated about his shoulder problems. When we asked how long he had been suffering, he said, "I've had shoulder problems on and off since 1999." I'm not kidding, you guys. Why was he waiting? Well, he did say he'd been to therapy here and there but it had never fully helped to get rid of his problem. Since he didn't have a terrible experience but nor did he have great ones, I can see why you may think all therapy clinics are alike. He was also relying on injections from his doctor, but the relief from pain didn't last as long as he expected. By the time he called us, 20 years later, he had lots of assumptions and experiences that held him back from getting the care that he wanted to finally get rid of his shoulder problems.

One downside of waiting as the problem gets worse is that it makes it even harder to confidently know whether therapy is even possible for what you have. It is possible to get the right kind of help with the right kind of program. We all need support to stay committed to

87

getting rid of the pain, healing the injured area, and having the best chance of keeping the pain from coming back. We work with clients who are as committed as we are to moving themselves toward their goal. We also spend the time to find out what it is that they realistically can accomplish with us.

Rose is another example of someone who is in the first group, having pain but waiting and not knowing exactly what is possible. Rose came in for shoulder problems after 15 years of waiting and wondering. One day, when she heard me talking about hand pain a light bulb came on. She said to herself, "ENOUGH!" She decided to get help for her shoulder (and hand) problems that had been getting worse over time. Rose is determined to get 100% better, not to stop at 80%. She knows after suffering for 15 years that she wants to learn what to do NOW in order to stay active and pain-free. She wants to make sure she learns what she can do to prevent this shoulder problem from returning.

We spoke about why she waited so long. She knew a medical doctor was not for her because they often prescribe medications or offer injections. She was scheduled for hand surgery years ago when she canceled at the last minute. She wanted to help herself in the most natural way, without pills, injections, or surgeries. She also didn't know who to trust. We were glad to be able to gain her trust and help her get better. She also recommended us to her best friend, who also started seeing us for a shoulder problem two weeks after Rose began her therapy.

Valerie is an example of someone who didn't wait long for help, but her journey was a little difficult in finding the right path. She is an active person who exercises regularly. Even when we think we are strong, there can be certain muscles that are naturally weaker than others. That is perfectly normal, even in people who work out frequently.

It's easy to have one wrong movement that causes the shoulder to "snap" or "pop." It's painful at first, but then the pain slowly calms down. You think, "Oh, I'm fine. It's all good," because you can move your shoulder. Unfortunately, after a few days or weeks pass, you suddenly feel that annoying little pinch in your shoulder. With the passage of more time, your shoulder becomes more painful with simple actions like getting dressed or reaching overhead to get something out of a cupboard. That's followed by more pain. Now you don't feel safe working out, or you can't get comfortable when falling asleep, or it's hard to stay asleep because your shoulder pain is waking you up.

This is what happened to Valerie, who came to our clinic with shoulder pain. At first, she tried to take care of it herself, but she was in so much pain that she was having trouble working and sleeping and putting her hair in a ponytail. She saw a doctor within several weeks of having pain, who gave her pills for the pain and sent her to therapy. Unfortunately, she wasn't making much progress in therapy, so he suggested injection, followed by surgery to clean out the shoulder. Her shoulder was so stuck and painful. But her MRI didn't show a tear of the tendons. She had a "frozen shoulder."

She became distraught over the idea of surgery. She did NOT want that. I mean, who wants surgery? She did not feel like she had explored all her options yet. She did NOT want PILLS or INJECTIONS either. She had already tried doing physical/occupational therapy, but it didn't seem to help. Frustrated and worried about possible surgery, she decided to try one more time with us at Hands-On Therapy Services, knowing that we help people like her to become pain-free while avoiding injections and surgery.

Have you tried going somewhere but were not satisfied with your care? This Miami woman wanted more one-on-one care and attention plus the hands-on approach to help her stretch and get rid of her pain. When she came to us, I spoke to her about what she had been doing at the other therapy center in order to explore what had worked and what hadn't. Most importantly, she wanted the one-on-

one time that we dedicated to her to get her moving. We used a lot of stretching and manual treatment to help get rid of the pain, obtain the motion she wanted, and get the strength to keep that motion and prevent further pain. Now she's back to her Orange Theory workouts – and we helped her AVOID SURGERY.

I did mention a third group of people, who were unaware of any problems with their shoulders. Then one day – BAM! They experienced tremendous pain and could not even lift their arm. Two clients, both named Marie, got help immediately because I knew them through family and friends. Both were relatively new moms with young kids.

As women who give birth, our bodies go through a lot of changes, and there are also changes in our activity level after we become a mom. There is a lot more carrying of bags, car seats, and the babies themselves. We put ourselves in different positions because we are breastfeeding or holding the babies. These are all factors that compound over time, until one day it happens. Both Maries woke up thinking they had slept the wrong way and could not – I mean could NOT – lift their dominant arm. They were in tremendous pain. It was constant and got worse if they tried to raise their arms. The worst thing about pain is how it makes you feel – frustrated at why it's happening, angry at how it happened, and feeling a sense of fear. Will the pain go away? How will I go to work and take care of my family if I can barely take care of myself?

Marie is a long-time friend of my brother. When she has medical questions, she trusts him to help her because he is a doctor. He was in town and invited her to our family gathering so I could examine her arm and give some advice. It was a weekend, so no therapy centers were open. Medications were not an option because she was breastfeeding. She couldn't even breastfeed her 6-month-old baby by herself. And forget carrying her 2-year-old, who still wanted mommy's attention and love.

The other Marie is a wife of a long-time friend of mine who is a physical therapist. He reached out to me for advice on something that could be done quickly. Who doesn't want to be cured quickly? There's a sense of desperation: "I REALLY don't have time for this!" Life goes on and kids' birthday parties are committed to and the kids still want to get out and play. If you can't move your arm, you cannot run after your kids, I promise!

With both these clients, I was able to give immediate advice specific to the trouble they were having. How could they position their arm during the day to have a little less pain? How could they position their arm for sleeping? Let me tell you, there is nothing worse than being in pain all day, feeling tired, yet not being able to fall asleep or stay asleep because of the pain. I was able to talk through what they could do to get some relief until we could see them in the office.

I would say that if you are thinking of a sling – or someone you know suggested a sling – please put it down and WALK AWAY. I know, your shoulder hurts and you feel like having something there to support the weight of your arm would take care of the problem. I promise that there are great uses for a sling! But when you have shoulder pain, as in these stories, I am telling you, the weight of the arm will pull and pull on your neck, causing even more problems in your shoulder and now in your neck, too.

Here are times you should use a sling: (1) If you fell and aren't sure what may be broken while you're waiting for X-rays or follow-up with your doctor. (2) If you just had surgery to your shoulder. The kind of surgery will dictate how long your need to use a sling.

Luckily for both Maries, they were able to learn what clear, actionable steps to take and get help in our clinic as fast as possible! At Hands-On Therapy Service, we have several options available to help you decide about your joint and muscle health, no matter what type of person you are. Sometimes we have people who have suffered a long time and just need to get started with our Free Shoulder Pain

Guide, providing actionable steps. You might need us as your second or third opinion. You can request to speak with us first to determine if we are the right fit for you. Lastly, when you are ready for the help that will allow you to be pain-free and active without pills or injections, we offer a free Discovery Visit. You can visit our clinic, meet the team members, and determine how we can help you. We want to be sure we can help before there is any commitment of time and money. There will be more about how you can work with us later in this book.

Actionable steps you can take

As specialized therapists at Hands-On Therapy Services, we are invested in helping you live your life to the fullest without pain or injection after injection that doesn't help. We take time to provide you with the information that you need both to live comfortably and to use your body in the way you want, without limitations. If you have specific shoulder issues but aren't sure what to do or not quite ready to spend time and money with us, then let us start with some actionable steps you can do at home.

- Have clicking in your shoulders when you are reaching overhead?
- Hear clicking or popping when working out?
- Wonder if something is wrong with your shoulder or could get worse?
- Want to know what the clicking in the shoulder means?

I get these questions A LOT. People are always asking, what does clicking mean and should I be worried? I want to ease your mind. NO, there's nothing wrong with clicking or popping of your shoulders if it happens EVERY ONCE IN A WHILE and without pain. It usually means that a tendon moved around in its space, which is normal. If it happens here and there with no pain, there's really nothing to worry about. Our body sometimes makes noises. Some people even "crack" their shoulder the way they "crack" a knuckle of the finger.

The biggest tip that I can give you is that if it clicks, pops, or cracks EVERY TIME you make the same movement, that's not good. For example, if you are working out and with every repetition it clicks, that is NOT good. Even without pain, your shoulder is telling you that something is out of place or there is a specific weakness. There is a rhythm to the way your shoulder moves, and if it's clicking every time, then your shoulder is not moving well.

Over time, parts of your shoulder can get tight, making that rhythm worse. That's when pain can set in and the shoulder can develop an "itis" like tendinitis or bursitis. That's when tendons can begin to tear. But if you are NOT painful yet, and your shoulder is just making some noise ...

- One way you can stop the clicking is to make sure you have good posture and position when reaching, lifting, or working out. Try to reposition yourself to reduce the clicking
- Stretches are GREAT. Make sure you have good motion in order to keep shoulders healthy and working hard for you
- Strengthening is KEY to keeping your shoulders strong and pain-free
- Massages can be great, too. Find out more about our wellness service specifically using instrument-assisted soft tissue mobilization for your whole body to make sure you stay pain-free and moving well. It's our style of "deep tissue massage" with tools, paired with stretching. We find all the good spots to work on in order to keep you healthy!

Is your shoulder already painful? Do you want to stay active and work out but are having shoulder pain? I have a story about Carl, who was referred to me by a friend. When his shoulder pain started about a year ago, he went to his general practitioner. He likes that they are a conservative practice that will give him advice on what he needs to do. Unfortunately, for his shoulder pain, they said it was most likely caused by arthritis.

He was directed to take medication and live with it, promising it would get better. However, his shoulder pain did not get better with pills. He went back to his doctor, who told him it was most likely arthritis and that he needed an MRI. It was something he would have to live with unless he wanted an injection or surgery.

His doctors did not recommend therapy. They wanted to give him injections. Although they said surgery was not a good idea, they wanted to do an MRI. An MRI is usually done to confirm what type of surgery you need. In our conversations he did not know that occupational therapy could help him avoid injections and surgery and reduce his pain, allowing him to be more active. Although we did not have a lot of sessions together (because he's from out of town), we were able to work out some of the pain. I gave him a few tips, one stretch and one crucial exercise to get him started.

Later, he texted me that he felt so much relief and was glad he came for a session. Though I was thrilled that he felt better, I was also glad I got across to him that he didn't need an injection or to take an endless number of painkillers or worry about surgery if he wasn't ready. I was grateful to let him know about more natural options available to him. Occupational Therapy/Certified Hand Therapy is an option for shoulder pain. He didn't realize that he can access occupational therapy without a doctor's referral as a more natural route to relieving his pain.

Whether you are feeling like Carl or your story is more like those of Valerie or Marie, here are some actionable steps you can take right now if you have shoulder pain. The tips below are for those who are having shoulder aches and pains, feel limited in what you can do, and are serious about getting the help you need to get RID of shoulder problems for good! If you are not sure what is going on with your shoulder, why your shoulder hurts during the lightest movement, or if your pain gets in the way of keeping active and doing whatever you want, then keep reading!

Here are tips on how any person who is living with shoulder pain can end shoulder pain and avoid it from getting worse. THE MOST IMPORTANT: come to our workshops to get more clarity on what's going on with your shoulder and so you can get to the root cause before you lose any more sleep tossing and turning (www.handsots. com/workshop).

1. **Don't sleep on the shoulder that hurts**. I know everyone has a favorite position to sleep in and that one of them could be sleeping on your side. But if your right shoulder is hurting, you will need to sleep on your left side for a while to give that painful shoulder a break. There's nothing wrong with sleeping on your side! I get that question a lot and everyone sleeps in different positions and often changes positions during the night. The problem arises when your shoulder hurts on your favorite side! By sleeping on that painful shoulder, you can make it more painful in the morning, make it stiffer, and cut off the blood supply that it needs to heal properly. If you are lying on your back for a little while, position a pillow or rolled-up towel under your arm. If you are trying to lie on the side that is not painful, use a pillow that you can hug, keeping the painful shoulder from hanging over your body. Get the help you desperately need to get rid of the pain and allow full healing. That will get you back to sleeping AND sleeping on your favorite side! If you need a visual demonstration, check out our Youtube channel as we have a video there showing exactly what you can do.

2. **Avoid reaching overhead**. If you are reaching overhead and lifting to put something away – or even worse, pulling something down that's over your head – AND you already have shoulder pain, you can hurt yourself even more. One of the most common shoulder injuries occurs when pulling

HOANG TRAN

something heavy DOWN. You can avoid injury to your shoulder by making sure that what you are lifting overhead is not too heavy for you to handle. Repetitive overhead activities, even though lightweight, can also aggravate an already painful shoulder. Normally, overhead activities are a part of what we want to be able to do. Try tucking your shoulder blade back and down, give it a gentle little squeeze back so that when you are reaching overhead, you are not in pain or feeling the pinch.

3. **Avoid reaching over backwards**. This is one of the most common ways that women injure their shoulder. It could be from reaching to grab their heavy purse from the backseat of their vehicle. Or reaching back to give things to their kids. OR reaching to turn on or off that lamp on the nightstand. You know the one move I'm talking about! A painful shoulder can result from over-reaching behind you. Adding weight to it from a purse or bag can make for a painful shoulder injury. I recommend getting out of your vehicle to get your bag or, if possible, leave it in the front seat where it's easy to reach. One simple trick that can help in the short run – until you get the help you need – is to slightly pull your shoulder blades back and down. It may help clear the bones from hitting each other. Where those two bones keep hitting each other is where people tend to develop tendinitis and rotator cuff tears.

4. **Don't do anything that causes more sharp pain**. Our shoulders do so much for us during our lifetime that by age 40 there can be significant wear and tear. One small thing from years ago can set off an imbalance that catches up to us one day. One of the most common injuries to the shoulder is a rotator cuff tear. Many people have small tears that happen over time but they don't even know it because it's not painful or limiting in motion or strength. Once you have pain with certain activities over and over, the best thing to do is respect your pain. Your body is trying to tell you something is not right inside. Over time, if you don't

listen, then you can completely tear that tendon, which may need surgery to fix. I want you to move, but you have to be more thoughtful while you have shoulder pain. Not moving is not an option, as that can lead to a frozen shoulder. Get the help you need to get rid of shoulder pain the right way so you don't have to constantly think about how you are moving.

5. **COLD versus HEAT**. If you have muscle pain, a cold pack for 10 minutes when you have the most pain or right before bed can help ease it. If you have shoulder pain because it's stiff, then you can use moist heat for 10 minutes before doing your shoulder stretches or while you are doing your stretches. Not only does it feel good, but it can help you relax so that you will want to stretch it more.

6. **Stretch daily**. Arm and specific shoulder stretches can help you maintain great motion, allowing you to stay active and pain-free! Stretches can be uncomfortable, and that's fine as long as you don't have sharp pain that radiates down your arm. After you let go of a stretch, that sensation of pulling or tightness should go away. Don't do a stretch that is so painful that the pain lingers. That could further aggravate the problem. Try doing some simple and gentle neck and shoulder stretches before bed. Just make sure to do two to three reps and really hold it for a good 10 seconds each time. Request our how-to videos by going to our website (www.handsots.com/end-shoulder-pain)

7. **Strengthen your arms**. Strength in your arms allows you to do everything you want in your everyday life and activities that you enjoy, too! Specific strengthening of your rotator cuff keeps your shoulder healthy and helps avoid common tears and injuries in the shoulder that can lead to pain and surgery. Strengthening is not the same for all muscles. Finding the weakest link and getting that muscle or group of muscles stronger is part of the solution. Finding the muscle that is working too hard and stopping it from overworking is also key to unlocking the full potential for

recovery. Key takeaways for strengthening weak muscles are that there should be no sharp pain, the muscles should feel tired (it is okay to be sore), and slowly increase resistance by listening to what your body is telling you.

8. **Give occupational therapy a try**. As occupational therapists (OT) and certified hand therapists (CHT), we are uniquely specialized to help clients with all types of shoulder injuries. So many people don't know how easy it is to access our services. You don't even need a doctor's referral or approval of your insurance either. The first step is just talking to us about your shoulder pain or stiffness that is limiting you from being active and pain-free! We invite you to come talk to us first so that we can determine if you are a candidate for our services. We also have amazing workshop events throughout the year that will give you an opportunity to learn about what could be wrong and get your specific questions answered. Nothing is more valuable than TIME, and we want to make sure that you get the most out of the time you spend in getting your shoulder pain-free and avoiding further problems.

I hope these eight simple ways to get shoulder pain relief at least gets you started in doing something, anything, to help your shoulder pain. Nothing is more annoying than when pain stops you from getting the rest you need or slows you down from being active with your family or from reaching your fitness goals! Whether you haven't tried anything so far or have tried other health providers, don't let that stop you from getting help to solve your shoulder problems! If you have tried something but your shoulder still hurts, let's talk first to see what is wrong! Then we can help you figure out the best solution for you.

If you aren't any of these people and are thinking, "I don't have any pain and don't have any limitations," then maybe you are like my Mary. I met her at a special event. While we were chatting, I told her what we do here at Hands-On Therapy Services to help our clients with arm and hand problems. She said she was lucky that she didn't have any big problems or pain. BUT she did feel achy or tight at the top of her shoulders and neck all the time, most likely due to a stressful job and being at a computer all day. She's very active and likes to stretch but was still tight all the time. She worried about the posture of her neck and shoulders. She was getting ready to retire and didn't want to develop problems or be unable to enjoy her retirement.

This is the BEST time to come to Hands-On Therapy Services, I told her! We have wellness services for people just like her, someone who is proactive and wants to learn more about what they can do and the best stretches or exercises that will help to release the tension and prevent injuries from occurring. The best part is getting the hands-on treatment to loosen all those tight muscles in precisely the right places. To learn more about our wellness services, read to the end!

Common accidents and surgeries of the shoulder

Accidents happen every day no matter how careful you are, and one of the most common is an injury to the rotator cuff, which are the muscles and tendons of the shoulder. These tendons are especially at risk due to their location and what they do for us. There are four muscles whose entire job is to hold and support the humerus (long arm bone) in the socket of the scapula (the shoulder blade). The tendons of these muscles pass in a very narrow area under the acromion, which is the bony part of the top of the shoulder blade. So often when I speak to people who tell me they have shoulder pain, they point to the ball area of the "shoulder." But the shoulder is made up of all the area around it as well. Due to the kind of work these muscles and tendons do and where they are located, they are prone to tears from injury or wear.

If you partially or fully tear your rotator cuff during a fall or while lifting something, most likely you will need a rotator cuff repair. If it is only partially torn, therapy is often recommended to seek to reduce the pain and strengthen the muscles to prevent further tearing. If it is torn completely, surgery is highly recommended but not a requirement.

Deciding not to do surgery for a rotator cuff that is fully torn is not a good choice unless there are other reasons like advanced age or a very sedentary lifestyle. Having worked with these types of injuries for many years, I would advise anyone with a torn rotator cuff injury to speak to their occupational or physical therapist that they trust and get clear advice on what they can do next. Surgery is a very personal decision based on what you want to be able to do – and whether you would be able to live with the consequences of not doing surgery.

I have a client whom I helped many years ago for hand and wrist injuries. She reached out to me because her shoulders were starting to bother her greatly. Her shoulder pain was interfering with her sleep and preventing her from being as active as she wanted to be. The pain was constant and driving her crazy. Turns out she'd had shoulder problems on and off for many years. She was at a tipping point. After trying physical therapy elsewhere without getting the results she had hoped for, and after having several injections, she spoke to me. I just tried to ease her decision. She wanted to have surgery and asked me if she was making the right decision. It's a hard and personal decision, I told her. I can't be the one to make it. All I can do is ask questions. Can you live with the pain? Did you truly try everything that you could to get rid of the pain? Are you prepared to do everything after surgery to get to where you want to be, active without pain and without taking pills all the time? Because it's not the surgery that's a problem. It's the therapy required afterwards that will be difficult.

Another friend of mine was in a car accident that resulted in a full tear of two of his four rotator cuff tendons and his labrum. We worked together to get the best motion with no pain. He did amazingly well, and because he could get to minimal pain and great motion, he decided that for him, at that moment in time, he did not want the surgery. He made that choice even though I had recommended surgery and spoke of the consequences of NOT having the surgery. He's still doing amazingly well.

When to start therapy after a rotator cuff repair can depend on the doctor's protocol. There are a few different types, and it depends on what the doctor likes to use. Generally, I like and recommend to the doctors who work with us to have the client come one week after surgery for passive motion and to be taught how they can start doing a few gentle things in the home. It also gives us a chance to help them reduce the pain and teach them what activities they can or cannot do after that type of surgery.

For example, after rotator cuff repair, you are not allowed to actively move the arm by yourself, which includes getting dressed or putting on deodorant or even your sling, for that matter. Some people are fortunate to have family or friends to help but not everyone and not every minute. MAYBE you were told by the nurse what to do and not do, but that direction was given alongside a million other directions. Going to an occupational or physical therapist from the beginning can help you learn how to safely move that arm in order to do your everyday essentials.

Another precaution after shoulder surgery: do not put weight on your arm, such as when getting in and out of bed. That requires put-ting to use the muscles that were repaired, and they are not ready yet. It's important to learn how to get in and out of bed without putting pressure on that arm. Oh, and don't forget positioning yourself in a comfortable way to get some sleep! How important is that?

Some doctors don't recommend therapy until after four weeks. During those four weeks patients are sometimes told just to sleep in a recliner. That can be even worse in terms of posture. I know when we work with people who have been unable to sleep for four weeks due to pain, they take much longer to progress because we must work so hard on getting the pain level down first.

My recommendations for sleeping after shoulder surgery is all about positioning the arm so that you are most comfortable to sleep. It is much easier to sleep on your back after surgery, although if you are not a back sleeper that must be torture for you.

"Do I have to sleep with the sling?" The answer is YES! Sorry, I know you didn't want to hear that, but yes, please sleep with it for at least a month. It helps to keep your arm protected while you sleep so you can't reach out and pull at the comforter or stuff like that. You can loosen it around your neck to you feel more comfortable if needed. When on your back, place a towel roll or thin pillow under the elbow area, not under the shoulder. The little boost from the towel just helps so that the arm doesn't "fall" backwards, and it helps the arm to be positioned in alignment with the body. It helps to ease the pulling on the front of the shoulder. Placing pillows or a bolster under the knees can also make the back more comfortable. If you are a side sleeper or have a lot of pain, this may be very difficult at the beginning. To sleep on your side can only be done on the NON-OPERATED side, and then the operated arm must be properly bolstered so that it's not falling across the body. I like to recommend a large firm pillow and position your arm so that is hugging the pillow while keeping your arm at your side.

If that's hard to imagine or you are a visual person like me, find Hands On Therapy Services on YouTube and watch my free video all about sleeping positions when you have shoulder pain.

After the first month of no active motion, you enter the phase where you start to move your arm using the muscles. By the third month, you can start to progress to strengthening those muscles. I can't stress enough how important it is to have a great therapist that specializes in shoulder therapy after surgery. You don't have to go to the ones that your doctors tell you to go to if they have their own therapy center or therapist. You can PICK the person that you trust to get you the best possible outcome after the surgery. You don't have to go to a place recommended by your insurance company. Insurance companies are concerned about not paying too much for the services that you need. The most important factor in finding your therapist is that you can trust them. Talk to them first and find out how much time and attention they are going to be able to give you. Find out what plan they say you need. We always like to talk to our clients before we all decide to work together. Having a specialist who has your best outcomes in mind will let you know if you are not progressing enough or at risk for complications. No one wants to have another surgery, so how you plan to progress in therapy is of utmost importance.

It is completely possible to get full recovery after a rotator cuff repair, though of course every case and everyone's body is different. What we do daily is different and how active we are is different. How we tolerate pain and how our bodies heal are different. Progress is not always the same from person to person, but you should be able to see and feel the progress with your trusted occupational/physical therapist working with you side by side to get you the best possible results. If you are not getting the recovery you had hoped for, read on to the end of the book to see how you can work with us.

Chapter 8

Cutting Through the
Questions After Surgery

Did you have surgery on you shoulder, elbow, wrist, or hand and now have questions about what to do next?

KNOW FROM TALKING to my clients over the last 20 years that there's always some confusion before and after surgery. It doesn't matter whether you have been mulling over a decision about surgery for months OR if you had an accident and now have a sense of urgency to understand what happened to you and how to rid yourself of your pain so you can get your life back. It can be so much worse when it's sudden and urgent, without time to think. Not being able to move, being in a lot of pain, and having many different feelings about your future after surgery is a lot to handle at one time. I want to help you get more clarity on what happens after surgery and the therapy you will need.

"You don't know what you don't know." That pretty much sums it up for so many of my clients when it comes to finding the RIGHT place or person to help them get the clarity and results they are hoping for after surgery of the hand, wrist, elbow, or shoulder. There is no crystal ball that will tell you the future. I often hear this in the way that our clients will say, "I had no idea that this was possible," or "I didn't know that I could have spoken to you before the surgery." You didn't know that you could get clarity on what is possible? That's why we do what we do at Hands-On Therapy Services.

Surgery is tough whether it is unexpected due to an accident or a decision you make to improve how you are living. There's a lot of pain, doubt, and fear. Understandably so. I've worked with other doctors, physical therapists, and occupational therapists who have had accidents resulting in surgery. Even THEY are fearful about reaching full recovery and doubt whether they are doing everything that they need to obtain the recovery they want. I've also experienced this. If health professionals – with their knowledge of how the body works – have doubts, fears, and uncertainty, it must be true for everyone who has surgery on an arm or hand.

Surgery is surgery. Lots of surgeons nowadays talk about "arthroscopic" techniques, but I can tell you firsthand that it doesn't matter how small that incision is, it still hurts. On top of that, you feel swelling like you can't move and start to wonder, "How am I going to recover?" and, "Is it even possible?" When you have surgery on your hand and arm, there are so many things that we take for granted every day.

One of my clients who had wrist ligament surgery after something fell on his wrist once told me how humbling it was when he couldn't tie his shoes after surgery. He had to ask his son to tie his shoes for him. He was taken aback as he looked down at his son tying his shoes, remembering a time when he had tied his son's shoes. Another client who fell and broke her elbow couldn't bend it to feed herself or put her hair in a ponytail. One client who had shoulder rotator cuff repair couldn't even lift her arm enough to put on deodorant. It's always the simple, humbling, everyday tasks that hit you first when they are suddenly difficult to do after an accident or surgery.

Once you gradually begin to do those tasks, other worries still keep you up at night. Depending on the accident or surgery, it can be life-changing. A long-time client of mine, Dan, was in a terrible accident involving his dominant right hand. He and his parents worried about what it would mean and how it might affect his life, his work, his hobbies, and his quality of life. Would there be tasks or activities he could no longer do? Dan was dedicated to doing the most that he could do to get moving. He became more active with his right hand day by day and week by week, without feeling limited. Years later I am happy to report that he is still active in running his company, playing sports, and living a healthy quality of life. He had been committed to doing everything he needed to obtain the best possible results from his surgery.

If you had an accident…For example, you're in a car accident, break your arm, and require surgery right away. You are being taken care of by many emergency room health professionals, including a surgeon you don't know and might not like or trust. Yet you are placed in a situation where you need to know and trust this person and others, as they are the ones who are going to "put you back together again." When you go to the emergency room, you already have an inherent trust that they, as doctors, will do everything they can to help you.

When it's urgent, there's no time to shop around. You get what you get. My client, Adam, who suffered a distal radius fracture after a car accident, was sent to a hospital where a plate and screws were used to stabilize his wrist (distal radius ORIF). After a follow-up visit, he was not confident about his doctor nor was he confident about the therapist who worked in the surgeon's office. He had many questions, but they were not eager to answer them or give him the time to ease his concerns and worries. Adam was not confident that he was getting better, and they had already talked about another surgery if he didn't make enough progress. He decided to shop around. He checked out several clinics. That's how he found us online and asked to speak to our specialist. He was invited in for one of our free Discovery Visits.

Shane came to me after an accident injured both his hands. Because he couldn't do anything, much less drive to therapy, he found us on the list in his doctor's office. Since I have worked with his surgeon in the past, his doctor recommended he see a certified hand therapist who could help him with his wounds and get him moving again.

When you have an accident that requires surgery, there are so many things that happen so fast and challenge what you know and don't know. After surgery, it's confusing with all the information about what to do next. Whether you are referred to the surgeon's own therapy clinic, referred to an independent clinic, or referred by friends and family, know that if you are not making the progress you need and want to make, it's good to ask questions and look for answers.

If you had an accident that does not require you to have surgery right away, you have time to find a surgeon that you know, like, and trust. You may accept the recommendation of the nurse or doctor from the ER. You may ask a friend or family member to suggest the best doctor who specializes in the kind of injury you suffered. If it's a hand, you would want the best hand surgeon, right? What if it's an elbow or a shoulder injury? You would want to find the surgeon who does elbows and shoulders all the time, wouldn't you? When there's a fracture or a tendon cut, there's some time but not a lot, so you are looking for who's good AND who's available to do you surgery as soon as possible.

If it's elective surgery, such as a partial rotator cuff tear, and you have decided that you can't live with the pain anymore, you may have gone to one or two doctors to select the one that fits you best. That's because you have more time to get to know, like, and trust the person who will perform your surgery. You might even have a therapy center that you have used and decide to let them try to help you avoid surgery.

Doctors specialize in medicine. Surgeons specialize in doing surgery. What happens after surgery? Occupational therapists and certified hand therapists specialize in movement to help you get your life back after arm and hand surgery. Most of the time, especially when it comes to hand and arm surgery, specialized therapy is required to get you the best results afterwards. The surgery may fix what bone was broken or what tendon was cut, but without a specific plan in place, not only will you be in pain and not be able to move, but, in the worst-case scenario, your hand or arm can get stuck and need another surgery.

After an accident and surgery, you will have a lot of questions. These are just the beginning of questions that you may have. In an instant, your life changes. "The questions are about the present and the future …your life changes," said client Rick, who fell and broke his distal radius.

Here are the TOP FIVE questions, based on my experience, that you may be asking if you are planning surgery or have already had surgery:

When Do I Get Started in Therapy?

There is a specific protocol for just about every surgery on the hand and arm. One of the most common misconceptions is that a person should not start therapy until after their wound is closed or their pain has lessened. I am a huge believer in the earlier the better for most cases. Since there are so many different start times depending on the surgery itself, my number ONE recommendation is to request to speak with a therapy specialist. Even if you don't know the name of the bone you broke or the type of surgery you had, by talking to you I can get a sense of what is going on so that I can make the best recommendation.

If you can imagine, a day before a huge hurricane was potentially going to rip through South Florida, we got a call from a worried mom. Her son had emergency surgery after his hand went through glass, cutting several tendons, nerves, and arteries just days before. Afterwards he was told by his surgeon that he needed therapy right away. The surgeon's office was one of the few places that provides a list of certified hand therapists whom he can call. Most people are told to go to therapy, but there is not a clear understanding of where to go, what specialist to see, and when to get started (even when told to go right away). What does "right away" mean to you, anyway, especially when your hand hurts and you have stitches from surgery? It's completely understandable because you don't know what I know when it comes to tendons.

I was able to speak with the mother and get a sense of where the cut was and what had happened. Just by speaking with her, we were able to determine that he had a flexor tendon laceration of many tendons along with the nerve. Tendons must be placed in a specific position depending on where they've been cut, and there must be an immediate start to moving the fingers in a specific way so as not to have any complications. We were able to get him in before this hurricane hit because we didn't know how bad the damage was going to be and how long places were going to be closed.

If you are NOT sure when to get started, call us or go to our website and request to speak to our specialist. And if you are not in the Miami area, you still can do this in your local area. The worst thing you can do is wait because you feel unsure. Sometimes we talk to people whom we discover are not ready yet and need to wait another week or two based on their surgery or injury. We just let them know when is the best time to get started. However, I highly recommend talking with a specialist, because most people benefit from getting started sooner than you might think.

When Can I Start Moving and Doing
Normal, Everyday Things?

This is a great question to ask your therapy specialist. Many times, when people are in pain and feel unsure about what is safe to do, they don't move at all. This can lead to more problems, such as getting stuck or developing complications in areas that did not have the surgery. The answer is to move what you can move or what is not strapped down after surgery. If you're not sure, call and talk to a specialist.

For example, if you had surgery for a wrist fracture, you can move your shoulder, elbow, and fingers. Or if you had a tendon laceration of your fingers, you can also move your shoulders and elbows, but you cannot move your fingers and wrist. If you had shoulder surgery, you might not be allowed to move your shoulder, but you can feel safe to move your hand and wrist, turn your palm up and down, and, in some instances, move your elbow.

Again, there are many different protocols. A specialist who knows what kind of injury and surgery you had can make the best recommendations. Sometimes, it hurts so much that people have a fear of moving. They often get stuck. We were working with a client after a severe hand injury. Because he had so much pain after his surgery, he did not want to move his elbow or shoulder, so he slowly started to get stuck as his hand became more painful.

I am a big fan of moving sooner rather than later. I have great relationships with many of the hand surgeons in the Miami/Fort Lauderdale area. I know how they do the surgeries and when they like to get started. I also am a big fan of connecting with surgeons whom I don't yet know well to get a sense of how fast they like to progress with certain surgeries. The surgeons can let us know how stable and secure a surgery is. From there, as the hand specialist, we get you moving, help you get rid of the pain, and help get you started on using your hand and arm in a way that can get you back to living a normal life.

Getting a clear understanding from our specialists what you can do and what you are NOT allowed to do is as important as knowing when to get started. At Hands-On Therapy Services, we take the time to talk to you before, during, and after surgery. We have videos from our extensive library to support you between therapy sessions. You'll enter a no-fail zone when you work with us, because your success is our success.

When Does the Swelling Go Away?

I want to scream the answer from the rooftops! IT DOES GO AWAY! I promise! It goes away. BUT you must be patient. I know that is NOT what you wanted to hear. I get it. I hear it all the time. All day, every day we hear these concerns from so many of our surgical and non-surgical clients. I hear that you are frustrated, have a sense of urgency to get better yesterday, and just want to get back to normal.

You are frustrated because it seems like the swelling goes away and then comes back. So this is my other most common question. "Does the swelling ever go away completely?" Yes it does. "When?" At some point MONTHS down the road, the swelling goes down. It does take time and may be one of the last things to go away. Some false beliefs about the swelling is that you must wait for the swelling to go down before you will be able to move, or that the swelling will go down only when you are completely healed. These ideas are simply not true.

Recovery after surgery is a process. You had an injury and then surgery. These two incidents cause swelling and swelling is a normal process of healing. There are ways and techniques to help reduce the swelling and keep the swelling down, such as positioning in certain ways, massaging, and using cold therapy. Movement also helps with the swelling as the muscles contract and help push the edema out of the hand and arm. Even when the incision is healed from the outside, your body is still healing itself from the inside.

When I was a therapist at the hospital, I once worked with this wonderful older woman from Israel. She lived there but came every year to Miami to spend three months with her kids. She fell while here and required surgery for her wrist. She got started with us between three to five days after her surgery. She was amazing in therapy. She was able to move well and did not have a lot of pain after surgery. Her ONE thing was that she loved to wear jewelry like watches and bracelets.

Both of her wrists were ringed with bracelets and watches as soon as she could tolerate wearing them. I remember she asked me if she should resize her watches because they still did not fit her well. I told her, "Ms. Brooks, please wait ONE year. I know it might feel like a long time, but sometimes the body takes that long to fully recover. You know scar tissue can take one to two years to fully mature and settle down, and after surgery your scar is not just on the outside but also on the inside where you cannot see it. Give it time to settle down and in one year all your watches should fit you again. Come visit me next year when you come back to Miami." Sure enough, one year later I could hear her coming down the hallway, all her jewelry clanking and tinkling. She came to show off her wrist in all its glory. You could barely see the scar, she had no more swelling, and everything fit like it had before. I often remember her as well as the many other clients I have worked with who ask me this question at almost every visit.

Remember Shane and Dan, who injured their hands and had surgery? Years later they both came to visit. All the swelling does go away for good. Which leads us to the next question.

How Long Is It Going to Take for Me to Be Normal?

First, you'll want to know when the incision closes and when you can get your arm or hand wet. It's usually the first sign you're getting back to normal and able to do the little things for yourself like take a shower, wash your hair, and get dressed. Slowly but surely it will become less and less difficult.

Then comes the harder part of asking yourself, "When will my arm or hand be normal again? I want to be able to move it like I could before the accident and surgery. I want it to feel like it did before the accident and surgery. I want to use it like I used to before the accident and surgery."

There are many of different kinds of injuries and surgeries of the arm and hand. I have seen everything from the complex accidents and surgeries to the less complex ones that you elected to have because it was causing you too much pain and lost sleep. No matter the severity, everyone after surgery worries and wonders whether it's possible to be normal again.

The answer for the most part is yes, it's very possible for you to have less pain or no pain, be able to move and function in your everyday life, and even get back to sports and heavier activities that you were doing before. I would be lying if I said it's easy, though. It's not easy. It takes a lot of work on your part. That's why we strive to be as committed as you are to getting the best possible recovery after surgery. So if you went somewhere else, and hoping for the recovery that you are not getting, give us a call and talk to us first.

I believe recovery has as much to do with having a positive attitude as anything else. Having great cheerleaders and supporters in your corner is a definite must. You know my two guys with hand injuries in the story above? Shane, who injured both hands, had amazing parents and family who helped him. Now he's doing great at work and even goes to the gym. Dan lives a busy work and play life after his hand injury, in which he lost a part of a finger. He plays squash, goes to the gym, and travels with his family and girlfriend every chance he gets.

Your life can get back to normal, too. Just know that it is never going to feel fast enough. You may even experience "heartbreak" or feel "depressed," words used by many of our clients in the past. Some injuries take a couple of months, and some take several more. No matter what, have a positive attitude and be persistent in the belief that recovery is possible. My longest-running client, Sylvia, has been with me almost 10 years. She was injured due to necrotizing fasciitis bacteria that affected both her hands and one foot. She was rushed to the hospital in the middle of the night with severe pain and swelling in three out of four limbs. Sylvia was lucky to be alive and to keep her arms and legs, but she had to endure a long recovery that required, overall, five surgeries to her hands. To this day, her hands are not "normal" due to the extent of her injuries, but nothing stops her! She is the busiest mother and grandmother I know. She probably does more now than she ever did before. You can find her at Hands-On Therapy Services several times a year to make sure she's taking care of her hands and arms so that they can stay as loose as possible, have less pain, and get stronger when they feel weak.

Anything is possible, no matter how long it's been since your surgery. It could be a few weeks, a few months, or sometimes it might take you a few years to find the right people who can help you discover everything that is possible, no matter what kind of surgery you had.

Do I Really Need This Elective Surgery?

This is a very common question, as it pertains to a specific injury or surgery. These questions are asked most often about injuries that are slow to improve, such as carpal tunnel release or rotator cuff repair when the tendon is partially torn. You just want to know if you are making the correct decision for what you need.

Surgery is a big deal. It takes time away from work and interrupts your family life. Not to mention someone is cutting into you. It's a tough decision for most people. Don't let anyone tell you otherwise.

Don't you want to feel comfortable with the decision that you make? I think it's very much a personal decision about for what's right for you. As with everything, there are consequences on both sides, whether you decide to have surgery or say no to surgery.

There are usually TWO reasons why people decide to have elective surgery: the pain is getting to be too much to bear, or the pain interferes with how you want to live your life. Ask yourself these three questions:

- Is the pain stopping you from sleeping?
- Is the injury stopping you from doing everyday things that you want and need to do?
- Did you try everything that you could using natural or conservative means?

At the end of the day, you must make the best decision for you. I hope that you did your research and had many opportunities to speak to your trusted doctor or therapist.

I have a friend who several years back injured his shoulder, fully tearing two out of four rotator cuff tendons. We worked together to get rid of the pain, and he was able to lift his arm, use it at work, and get back to riding his motorcycle without any problems. I recommended surgery in his case because he had a full tear of his tendons and is young (in his 50s). He may not be able to do certain activities as he gets older and will no longer have the option of surgery. He was able to do everything he wanted and sleep without any problems or pain, and he was able to do it all the natural, conservative way. He decided he was not going to have the surgery, and we discussed the consequences of his decision. It fit him best at the time. All I did was guide him by letting him know his options from the medical standpoint.

If you are talking with a medical professional about arm and hand issues, make sure that you become comfortable before making a decision. If it is an elective surgery, you have time to decide, and it is about more than having surgery or not having surgery. Don't let people make assumptions about you and what you want. Make the best decision based on the best information that you have. Talk to someone you know, like, and trust.

Important Aspects to Remember After Surgery

Never give up. It may seem never-ending, as you are going to have up and down days, but keep working on it. There is a light at the end of the tunnel. Consistently work toward your goals. You will be rewarded.

Go to someone who cheers you on and helps you over the humps. As you do the therapy, it's natural to stop when you feel pain. It's extremely helpful to attend therapy at a center where they help you overcome those barriers and encourage your achievements.

Keep looking if you are not happy or not satisfied. You don't know what you don't know, but when you find yourself in a place that doesn't value what you value, you will know that it isn't right. Keep looking until you find the place that will help you achieve the best possible outcomes. If you had a bad meal, you don't stop eating. Same goes for your therapy. Keep looking!

Attitudes play a huge role in your recovery. Maintaining a positive attitude and outlook is challenging when you feel limited and "depressed." Find a place that can help lift your spirits, allow you to have fun and be silly, and create an overall experience to help you keep going.

If you or someone you know are in the Miami area and planning a shoulder, elbow, wrist, or hand surgery, we have different options to help you get started. We understand that everyone is at a different part of their journey and needs different help at different times. Check out our website for free information, request to talk to our specialist, or apply for our free Discovery Visit. Call us now at 786-615-9879 to see how we can help you!

Chapter 9

Safe and Fit Living

O NCE PEOPLE FIND us after suffering for years with their arm and hand problems, they often wonder why they didn't think of coming to an occupational therapist/certified hand therapist sooner. Why hadn't anyone told them about this magical place called Hands-On Therapy Services? Well, to be honest, it's hard to act when the problem doesn't STOP you from doing your everyday tasks. People falsely think that because there is no pain... nothing is wrong! There are also a lot of assumptions being made about what you want, where you want to go, and what you are willing to do to get better. Sometimes you must try other things before finding something that really works for you.

I'm here to tell you, if you didn't know, that there is a **different way of doing things**! There is another way that you can get rid of aches and tightness, which will allow you to be more active and feel comfortable while doing the things you love doing. You don't have to wait until you have pain to fix your muscles and joints! If you knew that you had the best possible chance to avoid pain from stopping you in your tracks, and you were able to find a clinic that listened and delivered, would you be willing to try it out?

Therapy practice has been widely viewed as only having access under the direction of doctors and insurance. I can tell you that this is simply not true. It's a common belief and became common practice because that is how most people have used occupational therapy services in the past.

It hasn't been common practice to go to therapy when you are well, unlike going to a medical doctor or dentist. Most people are raised to go the dentist every six months and the doctor every year for a check-up. Occupational therapy is widely used all over the world but usually thought of only when there is a severe problem, when you can't move, or when you had surgery. **We want to be the experts you come to when you don't have major problems** – so you can AVOID major problems.

I can't tell you how many people we help with arm and hand problems who later tell us that other parts of their body are feeling tight or achy. Whether they came because they had an accident and surgery OR because they'd had enough pain and wanted to avoid surgery! At least half, if not more, tell us about other muscle and joint issues that they have been battling. If it's a hand problem, they eventually tell us about their shoulder and neck issues. If it's a shoulder problem, sometimes there is an underlying back or knee issue. We work with our clients to make sure we address the areas where they need the most help. First, we fix the hand or shoulder problem, and then we can address other underlying issues that have been lingering but haven't yet reared their ugly head.

We offer a maintenance program here at Hands-On Therapy Services that allows our clients to stay active without feeling so tight and achy. Taking your car in for a tune-up periodically helps make sure it doesn't break down on you. Your body's aches and tightness are your body's check engine light. Don't ignore it.

I'm sure you have heard from friends or family that it's okay if you are a bit tight or achy, that it's just something that comes with age or being active or inactive. It's almost socially acceptable to feel old, achy, and tight because, somehow, we are told by others that it's inevitable to feel that way. We are told to rest, ice it, or put heat on it. There are braces and medical creams sold by the millions. There are commercials about how fast and easy it is to get rid of the pain. **But therapy does not come in a pill.**

Something that sounds too good to be true – that you can pop a pill or place some machine on you and be instantly fixed – usually is too good to be true. It reminds me of a time I saw an infomercial about an electrical stimulation machine. You place it on your belly, wear it for hours, and suddenly you can get six-pack abs. I've never used such a machine, but I know that no machine will help you get a six-pack unless you are also practising healthy eating and exercise.

It's the same when it comes to healing your joints and muscles. There are no quick fixes for our nagging injuries. That doesn't mean that you need to come to our clinic multiple times a week (unless you just want to). It means that it takes commitment on your part and on our part to remaining pain-free and injury-free. If you want your muscles and joints to move and feel their best as you age, you must make that commitment to yourself.

We use several types of treatments to help keep our clients stay loose and limber, and we develop a program based on your needs. We provide a wellness service using Instrument Assisted Soft Tissue Mobilization with HawkGrips tools (check out what the tools look like at www.handsots.com/wellness and you can always follow us on YouTube or Instagram/Facebook to watch our stories). We pair our hands-on work using the tools with stretching in key areas that we know tend to be tight and cause problems. It's one of the best ways to catch a problem before it arises. For example, some of our clients with neck fusions or neck issues are avoiding surgery and need to make sure that other parts of their spine (such as their thoracic spine) stay mobile so shoulder and hand problems don't come up. Our shoulder clients come for our wellness service to maintain what they achieved in therapy and prevent another injury that could stop them from their activities. Those who have always felt tight all over love having a session to scrape and stretch out their back, hips, knees, and ankles as well.

Often people ask if this is like a massage. There are ways in which you can compare it to a massage because there is a lot of hands-on work. There are great massage therapists out there, but for the most part, if you are going to a chain massage spa or even a fancy hotel spa, you are there for relaxation. They massage your whole body and help you to feel refreshed and relaxed. As occupational therapists specialized to provide this service, we are like the mechanics for your body. Not only do we work out the problem areas in your muscles, we find the problem areas of your joints and how they move together to help you feel less tight, less achy, and less likely to have a breakdown. We are looking for your imbalances so that we can get to the root cause of potential problems and avoid having more pain. So, in a sense, you can feel relaxed afterwards, but the experience is much more active, since we move and stretch you to get to the root problems.

The imbalances of nagging aches and tightness that are created over time can start to become a problem. We use a style of treatment called Total Motion Release (TMR). It's how we find out where your imbalances are and help you fix them using our hands-on approach. Your body can be broken up into three parts: your arms, your trunk, and your legs. They all play a role in affecting how every part moves. Shoulder and neck problems are sometimes aggravated by back and hip tightness. Or your trunk being tight and not able to move in all its planes of motion can make your arms and legs feel tight. I always say your body is very smart. It will find ways to move so that you don't have to feel uncomfortable, but only for a little while. Over time, these compensations can develop into bigger problems. By finding out exactly where the problems are, we can move to fix these imbalances. We can also set you up with ways that you can fix it yourself between sessions. Our extensive library of videos allows us to follow up with you and help you be committed to keeping your muscles and joints moving freely, without aches and pains.

Many of our shoulder clients tell us about their back issues or leg issues. One of our wellness clients initially came to us after hand surgery and decided to try out our wellness program too. She had always dealt with feeling tight all the time. No pain per se, just tightness of her shoulders and neck and lower back. Another client, Ursula, works with her body as a performer, so after she came with her shoulder and knee pain, she decided to keep coming as one of our Year of Care Members to prevent injuries from stopping her work. Mary, whom you read about earlier, came for her shoulder but also comes for her feet and legs. She had surgery on her toes years ago but never had any continued follow-up. Now her toes are affecting how far she can walk. Our clients come for our wellness services based on their needs. Some come once a week, once every two weeks, or once a month. It all depends on what you want for your lifestyle.

We put our bodies through a lot when we are young, and because we were in our teens and 20s, the problems went away when we rested. Now that we're in our 40s and 50s, these problems don't seem to go away as fast. Our bodies experience a lot of wear and tear over time no matter what we do. Just like any luxury car that we value, we need to make sure we don't ignore the maintenance light when it comes on. We need to take it to a place that we know, like, and trust.

I also understand why people procrastinate in getting help for little aches and tightness. It doesn't seem urgent, but just because you don't have pain doesn't mean there isn't a problem or imbalance that you can fix so your muscles and joints support all that you want to do. Sometimes people tell us they waited because they didn't know that they can come to us first before going to the doctor. Most of the time they tell us they didn't even know this type of service existed. At Hands-On Therapy Services, we want you to know that you can come to us without waiting and that you can ask questions first when you are not sure whether it is appropriate for you now. We do what we do at Hands-On Therapy Services because we want our clients to feel confident and assured about what they want before spending any time and money with us. Read the last chapter in this book to find out how you can work with us.

Chapter 10

Why Occupational Therapy?

What is Occupational Therapy, anyway? What is the difference between Occupational Therapy (OT) and Physical Therapy (PT)?

WHEN YOU HEAR about occupational therapy or physical therapy, what immediately comes to your mind? What is your current understanding of what therapy can provide for you?

Most people I meet don't understand what occupational therapy or physical therapy even is, much less the difference between the two. That is completely understandable, regardless of whether you have had experience in therapy or not. Sometimes they seem more similar than different because, in both professions, we are here to help people with injuries or pain to get better. As Occupational Therapists, we can help you by getting to know where you are having difficulty in terms of your everyday activities of daily living, work, or hobbies. These are activities that you want to do BETTER but feel limited either due to pain or disability. We evaluate what you are having trouble with, break it down into steps, and help you to get to the root cause of the problem so that you can do anything you want to do without pain or having to take pills.

Not all physical therapists and occupational therapists specialize in the same thing or treat in the same way. Just like any other profession, you must find the place or person whom you trust to solve your pain. You have a lot of choices, and sometimes that can be even more confusing.

At Hands-On Therapy Services, we value time and attention. We understand that most people don't always know about occupational therapy or what we can specifically do to help them. That's why we give everyone we talk to as much time and attention as they need to make the best decision about who they want to help them with their arm and hand problems. In turn, the people whom we end up helping are looking for somewhere to go that will give them the time and attention BEFORE booking a paid session. They want to understand what we can do and how we can help them before they make a commitment.

It is not uncommon for us to talk to and help people who have gone to other clinics recently or in the past. There's nothing wrong with going to different places to make sure you are where you need to be in order to get the best possible results.

Do you think that therapy is somewhere you go only when you hurt yourself to the point that you can't move or only after you have surgery?

Occupational therapy is most commonly known for treatment after you've had a stroke and can't move your arm or you've broken a bone requiring surgery. While that is great and is one thing we do, we are also movement specialists who can help you to move and live again without pain. More and more people are looking for ways to stay active and pain-free as they get older. We are the best specialists to help you when you are just starting to have little achy problems that don't seem to go away on their own.

Do you think therapy will be scary and painful?

Since therapy is usually associated with an acute injury or surgery, it is often thought to be painful. That scares many people and deters them from coming.

Funny story: while I was with a group of other therapists for training, one friend who is a part of our group but is not a therapist asked for help with his shoulder. Something happened and he was in "agony," even losing sleep over it. He told me that another therapist was offering to do dry needling, and I had offered to help with my instruments. He didn't know what they were, so I described them as knives that we use to help ease the pain and get him moving better. He jokingly said, "Do I need to bring Band-Aids with me, because it sounds like everyone wants to cut and stab me." We can joke about it now because he knows us and trusts that we are there to help with his best interest in mind. However, when I think about my words and look at what we do, it's no wonder people are scared and unsure if we are here to help them or hurt them.

Do you think occupational therapists only stretch and massage you or use only modalities like ultrasound and electrical stimulation?

I ask because, before I can explain what we do at Hands-On Therapy Services, I want to acknowledge that everyone may have their own understanding about what occupational therapists or physical therapists do. Every clinic may have its way of providing therapy treatments. Many people have asked me if I simply massage or make them exercise, or whether I'll be using ultrasound, lasers, or electrical stimulation. These are all different tools in our tool box. As therapists, we do a form of hands-on work that feels like a massage to make sure we are working in the correct area to get to the root cause of the problem. We also use various exercises, done in a specific way to get you stronger so that you can be pain-free and more active. It's not like getting a general massage (which feels good and is relaxing). It's also not like going to the gym and working out.

At Hands-On Therapy Services, we specialize in developing a program that is specific to your needs. Nothing more and nothing less. It is not one-size-fits-all. Some people come to us because they like and want the hands-on sessions that we provide, and some people come to learn the best exercise that can get to the root cause of their problem, so they can practice on their own. Most come for a combination of the two. They come to discover for themselves what the possibilities can be to live more actively, with less pain, without the use of pills, and without injections and surgery. We offer a satisfaction guarantee, which makes it impossible to make a wrong decision. Ask us more about it.

Why is Occupational Therapy Better Than Rest and Pills?

Rest and pills may help you manage problems and pain that already exist, but, occupational therapy can often prevent you from needing unnecessary downtime due to pain and avoid surgeries in the first place. As occupational therapists and certified hand therapists, we are the mechanics for the body. Your body is the vehicle that takes you through life. For your car, you do things to take care of it, cleaning it, changing its oil, and rotating its tires. You are caring for your car so that it doesn't break down on State Road 836.

People commonly think you only need to go to therapy when something is broken. They usually come to us after arm and hand injuries such as fractures and surgeries. They come to us when they can't sleep and when their pain is too great. At that point they are like the car broken on the side of the road. They can't get where they want to go quickly.

126

Laura came to us for our wellness services because she knew that rest and pills were not enough. A friend of hers had come to us for our wellness services and thought that she could benefit too. She's an active woman in her 70s who loves to do yoga and play golf. She would play golf all the time if she could. She has always been proactive to make sure that she takes care of her body before it hurts too much. She came because she was feeling her shoulders and neck tightening up and felt stiff when she plays golf. Since being a part of our Year of Care Club, she plays golf more comfortably, without the stiffness during and after. She feels like she can get to the 18th hole more easily and even learned which stretches are key to keeping her loose. Since working on her arms and neck, we are also making sure her back and legs keep her mobile and free to play as much as she likes.

Resting is great, but, at some point, resting only stops you. Occupational therapy can keep you moving, problem free, and make sure that you don't break down.

Why Should I Go Here First Instead of a Doctor?

It's not that I don't want you to go to the doctor if you think there is something seriously wrong. I do want you to go to the doctor if you fell and think something is broken or dislocated. I want you to go to the doctor if you FEEL something is seriously wrong in your body. Who would know how you feel better than you?

I also want you to know that you don't have to go ONLY to the doctor. It IS possible to go to your occupational therapist FIRST when you have questions about your arm and hand pain, how you are moving or not moving, and how you feel limited in what you want to be able to do.

I spoke with James, who came in for his shoulder, who only found us because his girlfriend had started coming to us. He had a great opportunity to get to know us first because he would come to her sessions. He had questions about his shoulder. One of the things he told me was that he can do everything! He loves to work out but he was limited during a certain exercise because it hurt. After looking at his shoulder, I asked about his hands. I could tell by looking that something was affecting his nerves. "James, this didn't just happen," I said. "How long have you been having this problem?"

He told me it had been YEARS, but it didn't really bother him or stop him from doing anything important. He never went to the doctor because he felt like they would only give him pills or offer surgery, which he didn't want. James didn't know who or where to go to get the best answers for the problem that he was having in his shoulders and hands.

Only after working on this shoulder did we get the full story of what was going on with his hands. It wasn't because he didn't want to tell us but because he forgot. He's been living with it for so long that he didn't even think about it. He had no idea that he COULD access occupational or physical therapy services without going to the doctor. You CAN come to talk to us FIRST before going to the doctor while your neck, shoulder, elbow, and hand problems are just starting to bother you, when you are just starting to feel like you cannot fully do everyday activity or workouts without pain. Get peace of mind about what you can do to help yourself.

Why Should You Come to Us?

If you are someone who is having arm and hand problems, whether from a condition such as carpal tunnel or tennis elbow or an accident that required surgery, my hope is that this book will give you some clarity on what's POSSIBLE for you. It is possible not to be limited. You can be more active if you want to be. A chance to live and work and enjoy your hobbies with less pain and to be more comfortable in your body is within reach. If no one is explaining how it can be possible to avoid taking pills all the time and avoid surgery, I want to be the one to give you that glimmer of hope.

In order to do that, let me tell you a story. I was speaking with Maria, who works in healthcare. She knows a lot of therapists, and more importantly she knows a lot of doctors. So when Maria's hands started to hurt, she picked the doctor she thought was the best. And he's great. He's patient, gives you time, and is overall a nice guy and great surgeon. She went to him with a problem of her hands, and he discovered an issue with her thumbs. One hand was worse than the other. He told her that sometimes this happens to women and that at some point she would need surgery, but right now there's not much she can do. She said, "So I just have to live with this pain? It hurts, and without my thumbs I can't do anything!"

Your thumbs do half of the work of your hands, and when they hurt, your wrist hurts too, and eventually so do your fingers. It leaves you feeling frustrated and limited. It stops you from getting to do every-thing you want. Every New Year most people set goals and resolu-tions to do SOMETHING. Be more active or work toward fitness goals. As we get older, we must put a little more effort into what we are doing to keep our bodies strong and keep our weight under control to avoid health issues. I could tell she was frustrated that her doctor would tell her to continue suffering. How could NOTHING be done? I can't tell you how many people I talk to have been stuck there. They've been stuck there for years. It's not that her doctor is not good. He's great. He's a great surgeon. He knows how to do surgery.

As occupational therapists and certified hand specialists, we know how to help people get rid of their pain, get them to be more active, and possibly even avoid surgery or at least prevent it for as long as possible. For example, we helped Maria get rid of her thumb pain, taught her how to prevent and protect her thumbs from getting worse, and got her feeling like she could get back into activities she loves. She wants to stay mobile and participate in things like yoga so that she can hit her fitness goals of losing weight and feeling stronger.

That's why you should come to us at Hands-On Therapy Services. We are the ones who can provide you with solutions to your pain problems and get you to be more active without the pain and worry that it might get worse. We are the ones who can give you the best possible chance of not having reoccurring pain and tell you what to do if you do have something that does come back to bother you. This is what we will do for you that others won't: provide you with solutions that empower you to help yourself in the future.

How I Became an Occupational Therapist & Certified Hand Therapist

I've always been interested in healthcare because my parents always said it was what my brothers and I should do. In high school I volunteered at Miami Children's Hospital and was placed in the Occupational Therapy/Physical Therapy Department providing therapy for kids. My senior year of high school I chose to do an internship with the recreational therapy department at a psychiatric hospital. It seemed like it would be so much fun to play with the kids who were there or to run activity groups with the older adults who were there doing different projects. The occupational therapist there looked like she was just playing with the kids. Little did I know there was a method to the madness. I mean, who doesn't want a job where it looks like you are just playing all day?

When I went off to college at the University of Florida, I was between two different career options, but then I started volunteering at a hospital hand clinic. To be honest, I think I was only volunteering there because I needed to get volunteer hours. Lo and behold, I was really fascinated by all the different injuries of the hand and arm, and everything there seemed like fun. I would see the therapists make these cool crafty-like things that are known as splints. I remember one guy who came in with a snake bite. The poison traveled up his arm, so he needed a skin graft all the way up to his shoulder. I started talking to the patients, who would tell me some of the craziest stories about their hand injuries. They all had such great things to say about the hand therapists who were there. They told me how therapy in general had helped them through their different injuries.

I chose occupational therapy because I felt it gave me so much versatility. I could work with any age group. I could spend time with people, and there is a huge psychological component that I love. I could be creative. Most of all, I felt like I could have fun and help people have fun all while making real changes to people's lives today, tomorrow, and in the future. Almost 20 years later I still get to do that but even better.

All my training and work experience led me to love helping people when they are in their worst days. After graduating, I moved back to Miami and started building my career. In the hospital, people were there right after falls, illnesses, and surgeries. After moving into the outpatient department at the hospital, I still helped those at their worst after surgery or an injury stopped them from doing what they loved doing.

When I started in private practice, that's when I really started seeing the need for helping people in a totally different way. Yes, those who are injured and have surgery need therapy right away, and they are desperately looking for help. We are here to help them.

But there are also those who have been suffering for years without knowing what to do or who to go to because they didn't want to keep taking pills and getting injections and wanted to avoid surgery. I started to meet more and more people and LISTEN when they told me their stories. Not everyone wants to take pills and get injections or have surgery. There are many people who suffer in pain and are limited purely because they didn't know that there are other, more natural and conservative options to become pain-free and avoid unnecessary invasive procedures.

I've also had my fair share of injuries and been a consumer of the healthcare industry. I know there are other ways in which we can offer our services. I've been at both ends of the assumption story. "The whole prime rib?" I've made assumptions, and I've had people make assumptions about me. Now I've created a place where you can ask the questions that you want answers to without any assumptions.

You have many options for therapy services in Miami, and I want you to know that there are ways to get unstuck. I hope that this book sheds some light on the possibilities of living more active and pain-free. We do what we do to help serve you best and to help you make the best decisions about your arm and hands. So if you or someone you know suffer from arm and hand problems or have problems that don't stop you but make you worry about the future, then read the next chapter to see whether you can work with us.

Chapter 11

How You Can Work With Us

I F YOU OR someone you know are suffering with arm and hand problems, whether it's only occasional when doing certain activities or it's so painful that it stops you from living the kind of life you want to live, we are here to give you clarity about what you can do. If it's a friend or family member, please share this information with them. There are many ways in which you can work with us!

Who we help

We help people with arm and hand problems, whether you:

- Are tired of taking pills
- Want to avoid taking pills
- Want to get rid of your pain or annoying ache so that you can be more active
- Want to avoid injections
- Want to avoid surgery
- Had arm and hand injuries that required surgery

We help people with shoulder problems who have had issues for years, although that didn't stop them from doing anything, who suffered aches if they did too much or couldn't do certain exercises in the gym because they knew it would cause pain later. They knew something was wrong, but they didn't want to go to the doctor because previously the doctor gave them pills and offered surgery, which is not what they wanted.

Most people after the age of 40 can start to develop shoulder problems such as a rotator cuff tear due to normal wear. Those who have shoulder rotator cuff tears or shoulder problems due to an accident may require surgery. Getting started with therapy right away is key, as well as choosing the right therapist to help you achieve full mobility and the ability to use your arm without pain. It's a great time to talk to us to see what is possible, especially if you've been discharged from another clinic because your insurance benefits ended or your doctor or therapist thought you could do things on your own even though you're still having little issues.

We help people with elbow injuries that are severe enough to require surgery. Examples are a trip and fall, a car accident, and falling while riding your bike. Surgeries to the elbow may involve any of the three bones that make up the elbow or could be a radial head replacement, which means they replaced it with a new section of bone to make it into a new joint. People with elbow surgeries are limited in turning their palm up to wash their face or can't bend it all the way to touch their shoulder or reach completely straight. These are difficulties that impact how you can move for the rest of your life. So if you are not sure where to go first, or you are looking for more, then learn about our free Discovery Visits.

Maybe your elbow problems are not stopping you in your tracks like a fracture, but you suffer from tendinitis of the elbow. Whether it be tennis elbow or golfer's elbow, we realize it won't quite stop you from doing things. But I know from experience that it sure can slow you down and be extremely frustrating and annoying because it's so hard to get rid of. When you've been busy using your arms all day, you'll end up suffering at night. Talk to us to learn what's the best solution now and how to take care of yourself so it won't come back to bother you.

There are a ton of different hand and wrist injuries. Some result from using our hands a LOT. They are the tools that we work with daily. At some point you may develop tendinitis of the wrist, a trigger finger, or thumb pain. They can be painful, slow you down, and get worse over time to the point that you need injections or surgery. We have helped many people regardless of whether they come to us early. They may decide they don't want another injection and are not ready for surgery but are looking for a more natural approach to ridding themselves of pain and limitations.

Fractures of the wrist and hand are all too common. They protect us when we fall, and many fractures are bad enough to need surgery. Sometimes, not needing surgery is a good thing until the cast or splint comes off, leaving you stiff as a board. Cuts to the hand and fingers that seem so stupid can sever a tendon that requires surgery. All these types of hand injuries require specialized therapy after surgery for the best possible results. Not treating wrists and hands correctly after surgeries can result in complications, even the possibility of another surgery. It doesn't matter if it involves your dominant hand or non-dominant hand, most everyone we work with tells us their goal is having TWO working hands without pain. Whether you have hand problems that slow you down or hand and wrist surgery, we can help you get clarity on what to do next.

Our clients past and present also love our wellness service. It's our signature program that uses techniques to KEEP you moving without problems and without feeling tight all the time, as well as keeping you active. Therapy is not just for when you break down; it can be for maintenance so that you don't break down at all!

Why we do what we do

One of the reasons why we do what we do here at Hands-On Therapy Services is that we understand when you are in pain and having trouble moving you may be scared and unsure about what is wrong and whether it can get worse. This is a serious worry that plays over and over after you have surgery. It is the nagging worry that pops up in your head when you get frustrated or your pain reminds you it is not fully gone. This book is meant to inform you and give you some insight into what we do to help people with arm and hand injuries. We want to ease your worry, help you get clarity, and make you feel completely confident in the decision that you make about what happens.

If you did not have the best experience with other doctors or therapists, I can understand why you may be skeptical about how we can help you find a solution to your problem. It's like eating at a bad restaurant. When it comes to food, if you had bad Italian, you know you'd be willing to try it again at a different restaurant. When it comes to your health and healthcare, it is not so easy to trust that we could provide something different or treat you as a person and listen to what you need instead of making assumptions. We want to gain your trust first by making sure we can help before you make a commitment for a paid appointment. Not everyone is right for our clinic, and we are not right for everyone.

You have many options. Some choose to suffer a little bit longer to see if they can get rid of their aches and pains by resting. Some choose to buy over-the-counter remedies like pills, patches, and all types of braces (now they even sell pain patches that have low-dose electrical stimulation). Some chose to watch do-it-yourself videos on YouTube or watch on Instagram and Facebook various exercises that they think will help with their neck, shoulder, elbow, wrist, and hand problems. We work with a client who, after not being happy at another clinic, started watching videos on YouTube to try to get her fingers and wrist moving after surgery for a distal radius fracture.

We are thankful that she was only trying DIY therapy while she was looking for us. We also make videos on YouTube, Facebook, and Instagram to help those who are looking for a solution for their pain problems. JUST DON'T GET STUCK THERE! Don't get stuck using pills and braces and do-it-yourself videos when there is a REAL solution that keeps you from getting worse and not being limited in what you want to be doing. You ultimately get to make the decision about where and how you get help.

Ask anyone with an injury what they want, and they will tell you they want to get better as quickly as possible. Of course, they didn't want to have the injury in the first place! It's all the other questions about what you value that will determine what you will do next. I was on the phone with someone who injured his arm. He was told by his doctor to get started in therapy and was looking for a convenient place to go near his home or work. So I asked him, "Are you looking for a convenient place or are you looking for a place that is specialized and best able to help your problem?" He had not thought of it that way. Most people don't think of it that way either. One surgeon (whom I know and work with frequently) assumed that his patient wanted to go to a place close to her home and recommended his patient go to a hospital-based therapy center. They had no appointments for at least six weeks because they accept everyone, whether they show up or not. Thankfully, my client asked her friends and was referred to us by another occupational therapist. She doesn't mind driving a bit further for specialized care where she doesn't have to wait. I can't imagine what her fingers might have looked like had she waited!

We have many clients who start out with "I only want to use my insurance," and they are the ones who have used their insurance many times over without getting the results that they need and want. One man told me he has been having problems for over 15 years. He wears a brace on both his elbows due to the achy pain, but after speaking with him, he also had neck pain, shoulder pain, back, and knee problems. The pain doesn't totally stop him from doing anything, but he has used braces and taken pills for the last 15 years. He has also had a few injections that have not worked.

Apart the insurance issue, we want to have real conversations with the clients we work with. How committed are you to getting the outcome that you want? Because we are committed as much as you are committed. What are you looking for? We don't want to make assumptions about what you want and need. We want to know, and we work extra hard to make you feel that you want to come here because we can deliver on our promises when we both put in the effort. We have one client who very frankly told us from day one that he is busy and doesn't have time to do therapy on his own. In his words, "I'm too lazy to do it myself." That's a real conversation we want to have (without making assumptions), and now we can develop the BEST plan for the best possible outcome.

What we do

What we do is provide you with different ways to work with us. I understand that everyone is at a different place in their journey. Some people are just looking and wondering. Some people are more ready to act because their pain is getting worse. Other people need to make fast decisions, most likely because pain or surgery is stopping them from doing what they want to do.

We provide **FREE GUIDES** on our website if you are not sure what to do about your arm and hand problems. They are for people who are just starting to have problems, just want to see what it is, what they can do about it on their own, or what is possible. They are for someone who needs information at first, curious about whether they need to do anything, or curious whether they are already on the right track because they are trying to take care of it on their own. We get it. You don't feel the need to get on the phone with anyone right now. And we KNOW that sometimes you want the information but not any more than that. You don't want to be bombarded with tons of emails. I had someone suffering from shoulder pain tell me that at a community event. We hear you, too. You can grab your download and tell me you don't want any more information. We get a lot of other therapists grabbing our free downloads who will often email me after to let me know they are either a local therapist or from another state/country and wanted to see what we were saying. How cool is that?! So there's no risk in getting free information and trying out our tips. What could be the worst thing? That you try something that helped you? I would be ecstatic if you let me know that you tried something that made a difference in your life.

Besides the free guides that you can download, we also contribute by blogging weekly, AND we post videos to Facebook and Instagram AND longer how-to videos on YouTube. Look for Hands-On Therapy Services. Of course, you are always welcome to have a specific topic or video sent to you by email if you don't see it on our social media platforms or on our website. We understand that sometimes you are just doing your research. There's so much to sort through on Google, so ask us and we will send you the information you need.

For someone who's got a burning question and has already done the research but now needs a more specific answer, you can **talk to one of our specialists** at Hands-On Therapy Services. Been there with the Google searches, or been there at another therapy location, and now you are ready to get real answers for yourself? We want to make that possible for you. I often run into family, friends, and even strangers at the bar who ask me about hand and arm injuries. It's usually not just limited to that but also backs and knees (that will have to be another book).

Here is probably my most recent story, and I have a lot of stories! I was on a cruise ship with my best friend. It was great. I got to hang out with her, and we got to eat and drink. My goal was to finish writing this book. I am a talker. Outgoing, I would say. I'm sitting at the bar – anyone who knows me knows I like to sit at the bar. It's just easy. People come, are friendly, and start to talk and socialize. I met these people sitting next to me. They were singing along to "Piano Man"! How fun is that!? Of course, once I start talking this never fails to happen: I tell them what I do, that I specialize in helping people with arm and hand injuries. Larry's eyes and his entire body perk up.

"Oh, really," he says, "are you like a doctor?"

I say, "Even better, I am an occupational therapist and certified hand therapist, so I specialize in helping people before and after hand surgeries. I see that you might have a question for me."

"Oh, do you mind if I ask you a question?"

"Of course not!" I say. "I love talking and helping people understand what's going on in their hands."

He shifts over and opens both his hands to show me his palm, and I can already see what he's going to ask.

When you think about it, this is one of THE main reasons that I offer what I offer in my clinics. I can't meet everyone at a bar (for one, it's just way too expensive, and I can't be eating and drinking my life away). He opened his hands, and I knew that he had what is called Dupuytren's Disease. We spoke, and I was able to explain what it was and answer his questions. I helped put his mind at ease, because although he was still able to do everything, it was worrying him that it might get worse. It worried him to the point that he went to the doctor! We don't always want to go to the doctor! For him to have gone and asked about it meant he was worried. His doctor told him not to worry, that it was nothing and, if it got worse, he could always have surgery. However, he really didn't know what it was and just wanted to better understand what was going on.

After I explained it, he knew the name of the disease, and because he had a better understanding of what was happening to his hands, it eased the worry that he had going on in his head. He was thankful that I was taking the time to explain all of it.

No matter where you are in the world, and no matter what is going on with your hands and arms, I know that if you can get a little better understanding, you can make a better decision on what to do next, even if what's next is to do nothing and watch!

If you are in the Miami area and are ready to get a clearer understanding of what is going on with your injury or even if you are looking for a solid second opinion, then we welcome you to request to speak with our specialists. Get peace of mind faster so you can make the most informed decision. We will make recommendations based on what you ask us, and we're here to help you feel more confident about your decisions on what to do next, even if it's not with us.

Our **free Discovery Visits** are for someone who is ready for help, who wants to act right away. A Discovery Visit is a 20- to 30-minute in-person visit where you get an opportunity to meet and talk with a specialist. Our Discovery Visit is for someone who knows they want the help to avoid long-term suffering and needless injections or surgery.

It might be that you had hand surgery but aren't sure about the procedure that you had or when to start therapy. In that case, we invite you to our clinic so we can help you determine when is the best time to get started. Often we can help you get a better understanding of the injury or surgery you had as well. Maybe you are going to another therapy center or finished going to another therapy center and were discharged but are not where you want to be in your recovery. If you are looking for a second opinion, we can provide that for you.

Here is just one example of many. John was referred to us by another therapist because he was frustrated by a lack of progress. We invited him to our Discovery Visit to get a second opinion. He had major shoulder surgery and was facing a difficult recovery. Not all injuries are created equal, and his was a severe injury. We were able to explain things in a way that he could understand. I'm sure the doctor explained it, and his other therapist explained it, but it was not explained to him in a way that he understood at the time. We also were able to do a mini-session to see if HE could see and feel the possibility of getting better. It's always worth going to multiple specialists so you can be sure in your decisions. He came to us, and we were able to give him more time and attention, ask the kind of questions to get to the root cause of what he wanted, and explain it in a way that made sense to him. I can talk all day about tendons and muscles, but for him we needed to break it down and determine the specific things he wanted to do, such as being able to reach and shake someone's hand, which was really important to him. When we work together, it is possible to reach his goals and make his efforts worth it.

People who did NOT have surgery also apply for our free Discovery Visits. They are tired of trying on their own without being able to get rid of their pain and are ready to see whether it's possible to do something more to get better. They also want to show us what is wrong, where the pain is exactly, or what's limiting them when they move a certain way. Our Discovery Visits give them more certainty. We do a screening to see how they move, and sometimes do special testing so we can make the best recommendations. More and more people are applying for our Discovery Visit to tell us they have carpal tunnel syndrome or trigger fingers and are worried it might get worse. Those who we see and speak to can get tips right away about what they are doing right or wrong and start to make changes to keep it from getting worse.

Interested in meeting us for one of our **Educational Health Classes**? These are fun events that we hold at the clinic on different days and times. We get together in a relaxed atmosphere to learn about different problems that most people face or just to learn about how to stay healthy and fit. We talk, learn, and have coffee, tea, even wine depending on the time of day. It's a great time for us to give back to our community and help you make the best decisions about what you can do for yourself to stay healthy and fit. Find out more about topics, date, and time for our next events. Visit www.handsots.com/workshop

All we want to do is let people know they can change their story. We want to show them what is possible and what we can do together to make it happen. So the choice is yours. You can neglect your pain, stay worried or frustrated, or wait until you need surgery. OR you can go in the other direction and get some clarity about what's wrong. We do all this to ensure that you are someone we can help. It's our way of giving you a clear picture of what is possible for you. You need not continue feeling frustrated. The beauty is there's no pressure. At the end of the visit, you get better understanding about what is for you, and YOU get to decide what happens next.

I can't say it enough how proud I am of the team that we have here at Hands-On Therapy Services. We strive daily to make this a place where our clients feel welcomed, at ease, and happy that they are in the right place for the kind of help they need. If you didn't know, now you do!

FIVE things that we do BETTER than anyone else:

1. **We take the TIME to get to know you BEFORE you become our client**. You get to ask the questions. We promise to listen and answer your questions as best as we can. We want you to know the possible cause of what is creating the problem and why it may be happening.

2. **Get to the SOURCE of the problem.** Often the pain's location or the problem that brings you here is not the source. So often healthcare providers look at the one spot that's painful, but that may not fix the source of the problem. We want to help you for the now and also set you up for the best possible outcome in the future.

3. **We will see you for FREE first.** This is to make sure you are the right fit for our services and to help you feel confident in our services BEFORE you spend any money or time at our office. So often you are not sure who you can trust or go to for help with your specific problems – doctors or chiro or physical/occupational therapists. This gives you an opportunity to spend time with us to make sure that you want to spend your time and money with us to get better.

4. **You will always be treated with an occupational or certified hand therapist and given the time and attention you need.** Often, you may go to places where you are seen by the therapist at the initial evaluation but then passed to the assistant or techs sitting with three to four patients at a time. We want to pair you with the specialist that is best able to solve your problems, give you time and attention while you are with us, AND give you the support you need even when you are NOT with us – all to find the best possible outcome faster.

5. **You will become part of our family.** You know how you can always reach out to that best friend or family member when you need help the most? That's what we will be for you, once you are a part of our family. Call us, text us, email us, and use us as a resource anytime you have a question or worry. Now you don't have to wait and wonder whether something is wrong. Get the specialized advice without having to wait. You are always welcome in our house. We love it when past patients just stop by for some coffee. If it's at the end of the day, we may even have some wine together.

We offer many ways in which you can work with us no matter where you are in your journey. We are also proud of the "fail-proof" environment that we have created for you to feel safe in doing business with us. Ask us about our Satisfaction Guarantee. If we can give you just an ounce of ease or clarity for you to make the best decision, then we are happy to know that we made a difference. If you or someone you know is suffering and feeling unsure about their arm and hand problems, please consider sharing this book and check us out online at www.handsots.com so that you can get some answers and peace of mind! Thank you for allowing me to help you on this journey we call LIVING!

Find **Hands-On Therapy Services**
online at **www.handsots.com**

Follow and subscribe on YouTube,
Instagram, and Facebook

Made in the USA
Coppell, TX
09 July 2020